Advanced Lung Cancer: Radical Surgical Therapy

Editor

RAJA M. FLORES

THORACIC SURGERY CLINICS

www.thoracic.theclinics.com

Consulting Editor
M. BLAIR MARSHALL

November 2014 • Volume 24 • Number 4

ELSEVIER

1600 John F. Kennedy Boulevard • Suite 1800 • Philadelphia, Pennsylvania, 19103-2899

http://www.thoracic.theclinics.com

THORACIC SURGERY CLINICS Volume 24, Number 4
November 2014 ISSN 1547-4127, ISBN-13: 978-0-323-32389-5

Editor: John Vassallo (j.vassallo@elsevier.com)
Developmental Editor: Stephanie Carter

Thoracic Surgery Clinics (ISSN 1547-4127) is published quarterly by Elsevier Inc., 360 Park Avenue South, New York, NY 10010-1710. Months of publication are February, May, August, and November. Business and editorial offices: 1600 John F. Kennedy Boulevard, Suite 1800, Philadelphia, PA 19103-2899. Periodicals postage paid at New York, NY, and additional mailing offices. Subscription prices are $350.00 per year (US individuals), $453.00 per year (US institutions), $165.00 per year (US Students), $435.00 per year (Canadian individuals), $585.00 per year (Canadian institutions), $225.00 per year (Canadian and foreign students), $465.00 per year (foreign individuals), and $585.00 per year (foreign institutions). Foreign air speed delivery is included in all Clinics' subscription prices. All prices are subject to change without notice. **POSTMASTER:** Send address changes to Thoracic Surgery Clinics, Elsevier Health Sciences Division, Subscription Customer Service, 3251 Riverport Lane, Maryland Heights, MO 63043. **Customer Service (orders, claims, online, change of address): Telephone: 1-800-654-2452 (U.S. and Canada); 314-447-8871 (outside U.S. and Canada). Fax: 314-447-8029. E-mail: journalscustomerservice-usa@elsevier.com (for print support); journalsonlinesupport-usa@elsevier.com (for online support).**

Reprints. For copies of 100 or more, of articles in this publication, please contact Commercial Rights Department, Elsevier Inc., 360 Park Avenue South, New York, NY 10010-1710. Tel: 212-633-3874; Fax: 212-633-3820; E-mail: reprints@elsevier.com.

Thoracic Surgery Clinics is covered in *MEDLINE/PubMed (Index Medicus), EMBASE/Excerpta Medica, Science Citation Index Expanded (SciSearch®), Journal Citation Reports/Science Edition,* and *Current Contents®/Clinical Medicine.*

Contributors

CONSULTING EDITOR

M. BLAIR MARSHALL, MD, FACS
Chief, Division of Thoracic Surgery; Associate
Professor of Surgery, Department of Surgery,
Georgetown University Medical Center,
Georgetown University School of Medicine,
Washington, DC

EDITOR

RAJA M. FLORES, MD
Ames Professor of Cardiothoracic Surgery;
Chairman, Department of Thoracic Surgery
Mount Sinai Health System, Icahn School of
Medicine at Mount Sinai New York, New York

AUTHORS

NAVEED ZEB ALAM, MD, FRCSC, FRACS
Consultant Thoracic Surgeon and Senior
Lecturer, St Vincent's Hospital, University of
Melbourne, Melbourne, Victoria, Australia

KATHERINE W. ARMSTRONG, MPH
Project Manager, Division of Thoracic Surgery,
Brigham and Women's Hospital, Harvard
Medical School, Boston, Massachusetts

DANIEL BARALE, MD
Thoracic Surgery, University Hospital Careggi,
Florence, Italy

DAINE T. BENNETT, MD
Surgical Resident, Division of Cardiothoracic
Surgery, Department of Surgery, University of
Colorado Denver, School of Medicine, Aurora,
Colorado

MARK H. BILSKY, MD
Department of Neurosurgery, Memorial
Sloan-Kettering Cancer Center, New York,
New York

CARLOS BRAVO-IÑIGUEZ, MD
Research Fellow, Division of Thoracic Surgery,
Brigham and Women's Hospital, Harvard
Medical School, Boston, Massachusetts

ANTONIO D'ANDRILLI, MD
Assistant Professor of Thoracic Surgery,
Department of Thoracic Surgery, Sant'Andrea
Hospital, University LaSapienza, Rome, Italy

ALBERTO DE HOYOS, MD, FACS, FCCP
Associate Professor of Surgery; Director,
Minimally Invasive and Robotic Thoracic
Surgery, Northwestern Memorial Hospital,
Northwestern University Feinberg School of
Medicine, Chicago, Illinois

MARC DE PERROT, MD
Division of Thoracic Surgery, Toronto General
Hospital, University Health Network, University
of Toronto, Toronto, Ontario, Canada

MALCOLM M. DeCAMP, MD, FACS, FCCP
Fowler McCormick Professor of Surgery; Chief,
Division of Thoracic Surgery, Northwestern
Memorial Hospital, Northwestern University
Feinberg School of Medicine, Chicago, Illinois

JESSICA S. DONINGTON, MD
Associate Professor, Department of
Cardiothoracic Surgery; Director of Thoracic
Surgery, Bellevue Hospital, NYU School of
Medicine, New York, New York

ROBERT J. DOWNEY, MD
Professor of Surgery, Thoracic Service,
Department of Surgery, Memorial Hospital,
Memorial Sloan Kettering Cancer Center,
New York, New York

RAJA M. FLORES, MD
Professor and Chairman, Department of
Thoracic Surgery, Mount Sinai Health System,
Icahn School of Medicine at Mount Sinai,
New York, New York

ALESSANDRO GONFIOTTI, MD
Thoracic Surgery, University Hospital Careggi,
Florence, Italy

MICHAEL THOMAS JAKLITSCH, MD
Associate Professor of Surgery; Surgeon,
Division of Thoracic Surgery, Brigham and
Women's Hospital, Harvard Medical School,
Boston, Massachusetts

MASSIMO OSVALDO JAUS, MD
General and Thoracic Surgery, Sandro Pertini
Hospital, Rome, Italy

STEFAN S. KACHALA, MD
Department of Thoracic and Cardiovascular
Surgery, Cleveland Clinic, Cleveland, Ohio

SHAF KESHAVJEE, MD, FRCSC, FACS
Professor, Division of Thoracic Surgery;
Professor, Institute of Biomaterials and
Bioengineering, Toronto General Hospital,
University Health Network, University of
Toronto, Toronto, Ontario, Canada

ILYA LAUFER, MD
Department of Neurosurgery, Memorial
Sloan-Kettering Cancer Center, New York,
New York

DONG-SEOK D. LEE, MD
Assistant Professor, Department of Thoracic
Surgery, Mount Sinai Health System, Icahn
School of Medicine at Mount Sinai, New York,
New York

PAOLO MACCHIARINI, MD, PhD
Advanced Center for Translational
Regenerative Medicine (ACTREM), Karolinska
Institutet, Stockholm, Sweden

MAURICIO PEREZ MARTINEZ, MD
Research Fellow, Division of Thoracic Surgery,
Brigham and Women's Hospital, Harvard
Medical School, Boston, Massachusetts

EVAN MATROS, MD
Plastic Surgery Service, Department of
Surgery, Memorial Sloan-Kettering Cancer
Center, New York, New York

GIULIO MAURIZI, MD
Resident of Thoracic Surgery, Department of
Thoracic Surgery, Sant'Andrea Hospital,
University LaSapienza, Rome, Italy

OLAF MERCIER, MD
Division of Thoracic Surgery, Toronto General
Hospital, University Health Network, University
of Toronto, Toronto, Ontario, Canada

NATHAN M. MOLLBERG, DO
Division of Cardiothoracic Surgery,
Department of Surgery, University of
Washington, Seattle, Washington

MICHAEL S. MULLIGAN, MD
Division of Cardiothoracic Surgery,
Department of Surgery, University of
Washington, Seattle, Washington

SUDISH C. MURTHY, MD, PhD
Section Head, Thoracic Surgery, Department
of Thoracic and Cardiovascular Surgery,
Cleveland Clinic, Cleveland, Ohio

HARVEY I. PASS, MD
Division Chief, General Thoracic Surgery;
Stephen E. Banner Professor of Thoracic
Oncology, Vice-Chair Research, Department of
Cardiothoracic Surgery, NYU Langone Medical
Center, NYU School of Medicine, New York,
New York

EMILY S. REARDON, MD
Thoracic Surgery Section, Thoracic and GI
Oncology Branch, CCR/NCI, National
Institutes of Health, Bethesda, Maryland

ERINO A. RENDINA, MD
Professor and Chief, Department of Thoracic
Surgery, Sant'Andrea Hospital, University
LaSapienza; Spencer-Cenci Foundation,
Rome, Italy

VALERIE W. RUSCH, MD
Thoracic Surgery Service, Department of
Surgery, Memorial Sloan-Kettering Cancer
Center, New York, New York

DAVID S. SCHRUMP, MD, MBA
Thoracic Surgery Section, Senior Investigator
and Surgical Chief, Thoracic and GI Oncology
Branch, CCR/NCI, National Institutes of Health,
Bethesda, Maryland

FEDERICO VENUTA, MD
Professor and Chief, Department of Thoracic
Surgery, Policlinico Umberto I, University
LaSapienza; Spencer-Cenci Foundation,
Rome, Italy

MICHAEL J. WEYANT, MD
Associate Professor of Surgery, Section of
General Thoracic Surgery, Division of
Cardiothoracic Surgery, University of Colorado
Denver, School of Medicine, Aurora, Colorado

ANDREA S. WOLF, MD
Professor and Surgeon, Department of
Thoracic Surgery, Mount Sinai Health System,
Icahn School of Medicine at Mount Sinai,
New York, New York

JOSHUA YAMADA, MD
Department of Radiation Oncology, Memorial
Sloan-Kettering Cancer Center, New York,
New York

FEDERICO VENUTA, MD
Professor and Chief, Department of Thoracic Surgery, Policlinico Umberto I, University LaSapienza; Spencer Cenci Foundation, Rome, Italy

MICHAEL J. WEYANT, MD
Associate Professor of Surgery, Section of General Thoracic Surgery, Division of Cardiothoracic Surgery, University of Colorado Denver, School of Medicine, Aurora, Colorado

ANDREA S. WOLF, MD
Professor and Surgeon, Department of Thoracic Surgery, Mount Sinai Health System, Icahn School of Medicine at Mount Sinai, New York, New York

JOSHUA YAMADA, MD
Department of Radiation Oncology, Memorial Sloan-Kettering Cancer Center, New York, New York

Contents

> An overview of preoperative risk assessment in marginal patients being considered for surgical resection with curative intent for non–small cell lung cancer is provided. The examination of modifiers of standard risk models including surgical approach, specific anatomic considerations, and the use of lung-sparing techniques is discussed.

> Assessment for thoracic surgery in elderly patients should be based on physiologic rather than chronologic age. Thoracic surgery offers the best chance for cure in patients with early-stage lung cancer, and has been shown to be safe in carefully selected candidates. A targeted preoperative assessment can help individualize the risk of morbidity and mortality for each patient, and thus provide both surgeon and patient with the information needed for operative decision making.

> Resection of the chest wall for lung cancer by definition indicates locally advanced disease. Complete en bloc removal of the tumor and thorough surgical staging is paramount for offering the best treatment and increasing the chances of prolonged survival. Thorough knowledge of all the reconstructive techniques available is critical to allow appropriate operative planning. A multidisciplinary approach including involvement of plastic and spinal surgery expertise should be considered when planning a large resection. Repairs should give structural stability while maintaining functional capacity of the thorax. Respiratory and wound complications are the most frequent postoperative issues.

> Multiple retrospective studies suggest that there may be a survival benefit to surgical resection of the primary site of a non–small cell lung cancer (NSCLC) and of a single (oligometastatic) M1 site of disease. There is only one published nonrandomized trial addressing the effectiveness of surgical resection of the primary site and an M1 site of NSCLC, which did not show a benefit of adding surgery to systemic chemotherapy. Prospective trials are likely to be difficult to complete because of multiple factors; possible trial designs are suggested.

Small-cell lung cancer (SCLC) comprises approximately 14% of all lung cancer cases. Most patients present with locally advanced or metastatic disease and are therefore treated nonoperatively with chemotherapy, radiotherapy, or both. A small subset of patients with SCLC present with early-stage disease and will benefit from surgical resection plus chemotherapy. The rationale for radiotherapy in these patients remains controversial.

Lobectomy with reconstruction of the bronchus and pulmonary artery is a viable therapeutic option for patients with centrally located non–small cell lung cancer. Preoperative chemotherapy or chemoradiotherapy may represent an additional risk factor for postoperative complications because of increased difficulty in surgical dissection and potential impairment of bronchial healing. Although limited data are available in the literature in this setting, a few published studies have reported the possibility of performing even complex bronchovascular reconstructions after neo-adjuvant treatment with no increased morbidity and mortality. This article discusses the main technical details and data from the literature.

The management of NSCLC involving the spine has evolved significantly during the past decade. Current treatment is based on MRI findings and combined evaluation of neurologic, oncologic, mechanical, and systemic (NOMS) disease issues. Advances in radiotherapy now permit effective treatment of spinal lesions previously managed surgically. Conversely, improvements in hardware now allow better stabilization of the spine and early mobilization of patients who require surgical intervention.

Patients who develop a second primary lung cancer after pneumonectomy may benefit from an additional resection and should not be automatically excluded from surgical consideration. These patients should be carefully selected based on lung cancer stage and cardiopulmonary reserve. The most important initial differentiation is to distinguish a true second primary lung cancer from metastatic recurrent lung cancer. Only patients who have stage I disease are candidates for this type of extended resection. Wedge resection with negative margins is the preferred procedure for peripheral tumors. Central tumors are effectively treated with segmentectomy.

Invasion of the superior vena cava (SVC) by lung cancer is no longer deemed unresectable. Patient presentation and patterns of involvement are heterogeneous. Careful preoperative evaluation is necessary to determine resectability. Partial or complete SVC resection may be required, and reconstruction may be accomplished with suture repair, patch repair, or prosthesis, with acceptable short- and long-term outcomes.

Jessica S. Donington and Harvey I. Pass

The treatment algorithm for locally advanced non–small cell lung cancer is complex and may best be described as chemotherapy-based multimodality therapy, but there is little consensus as to what constitutes the optimal approach to localized therapy in this setting. The extent of mediastinal lymph node involvement is the principal factor dictating the benefit that can be derived from resection. Surgery is reserved for those with occult N2 disease or discrete resectable N2 involvement. Debate exists over which patients with potentially resectable N2 should undergo resection and how to best integrate resection with chemotherapy and radiation.

Emily S. Reardon and David S. Schrump

Historically, extended resections for T4 non-small cell lung cancers that invade adjacent organs have been associated with significant morbidity and mortality, and poor long-term survival. However, notable improvements in imaging, surgical techniques, and perioperative care during the past several decades have resulted in an increase in survival for highly selected patients. This article provides a critical review of the existing statistical evidence regarding the utility of resections of T4 tumors invading the aorta, pulmonary artery, left atrium, and esophagus.

Nathan M. Mollberg and Michael S. Mulligan

Concerns regarding the sequelae of neoadjuvant chemotherapy or chemoradiotherapy on the pleural space and tissue planes had previously deterred the application of video-assisted thoracoscopic (VATS) lobectomy for patients who underwent neoadjuvant therapy. As experience with VATS has increased, however, its application toward more technically demanding operations has also expanded. The diminished impact on pulmonary function associated with the VATS approach may make pulmonary resection more tolerable in compromised patients. This article describes an approach designed for maximal safety on carefully selected patients who have undergone induction therapy.

Andrea S. Wolf and Raja M. Flores

Although most commonly associated with surgery for malignant pleural mesothelioma, extrapleural pneumonectomy (EPP) may be used to treat patients with pleural dissemination of other malignancies. Patients who present with stage IV nonsmall cell lung cancer (NSCLC) caused by malignant pleural effusion may be considered for EPP following induction chemotherapy if they demonstrate no mediastinal nodal or distant metastases and have adequate cardiopulmonary reserve. With careful preoperative evaluation and perioperative care, the rates of complication and/or death are acceptable. Nevertheless, EPP for NSCLC should be performed by experienced teams at experienced centers to minimize morbidity and mortality.

THORACIC SURGERY CLINICS

RELATED INTEREST

Radiologic Clinics of North America, Volume 52, Issue 1 (January 2014)
Thoracic Imaging
Jane P. Ko, *Editor*
Available at: www.radiology.theclinics.com

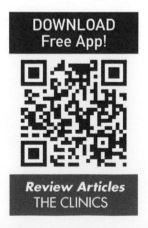

NOW AVAILABLE FOR YOUR iPhone and iPad

Preface
Advanced Lung Cancer: Radical Surgical Therapy

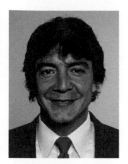

Raja M. Flores, MD
Editor

Advanced lung cancer is synonymous with patients suffering from stage III and IV disease. Surgery is not routinely recommended for patients with such advanced disease and must be evaluated on a case-by-case basis. Many times this is a personal choice for the patient. Younger and stronger patients tend to seek out more aggressive therapy. This issue was designed as a resource for surgeons treating patients seeking radical surgical treatment.

Advancements in chemotherapy and targeted therapy have influenced our decisions to perform procedures that we normally would not consider in our surgical repertoire for routine treatment. The older definition of radical surgery meant removing the mediastinal lymph nodes with either a lobectomy or a pneumonectomy. Today, radical surgery implies resection of structures adjacent to the lung that would normally not be resected in an effort to obtain negative margins. Radical surgery also encompasses resection in patients otherwise deemed too high-risk for surgery based on physiologic factors, metastasis of cancer, or extent of resection.

The decision to operate on such cases requires evaluation of tumor biology, assessment of response to neoadjuvant therapy, careful surgical planning, and an in-depth dialogue with the patient to ensure a realistic view of the possible outcomes.

The articles in this issue are written by many distinguished surgeons who have first-hand experience in performing these procedures. Surgical technique is critical; however, careful patient selection is the key to successful outcomes.

Raja M. Flores, MD
Ames Professor of Cardiothoracic Surgery
Chairman, Department of Thoracic Surgery
Mount Sinai Health System
Icahn School of Medicine at Mount Sinai
One Gustave L. Levy Place, Box 1023
New York, NY 10029, USA

E-mail address:
Raja.Flores@mountsinai.org

Thorac Surg Clin 24 (2014) xiii
http://dx.doi.org/10.1016/j.thorsurg.2014.08.002
1547-4127/14/$ – see front matter © 2014 Elsevier Inc. All rights reserved.

Erratum

In the August 2014 issue (Volume 24, number 3), the article "Peptide Receptor Radionuclide Therapy for Advanced Neuroendocrine Tumors," lists co-author Giovanni Paganelli's dual affiliation incorrectly. His correct affiliation is: Giovanni Paganelli, MD, Radiometabolic Unit, Department of Nuclear Medicine, Istituto Scientifico Romagnolo per lo Studio e la Cura dei Tumori (IRST), IRCCS, Meldola, Italy.

http://dx.doi.org/10.1016/j.thorsurg.2014.09.003
1547-4127/14/$ – see front matter

Erratum

In the August 2014 issue (Volume 24, number 3), the article "Peptide Receptor Radionuclide Therapy for Advanced Neuroendocrine Tumors." lists co-author Giovanni Paganelli's dual affiliation incorrectly. His correct affiliation is Giovanni Paganelli, MD, Radiometabolic Unit, Department of Nuclear Medicine, Istituto Scientifico Romagnolo per lo Studio e la Cura dei Tumori (IRST), IRCCS, Meldola, Italy.

Lung Resection in Patients with Marginal Pulmonary Function

Naveed Zeb Alam, MD, FRCSC, FRACS

KEYWORDS

- Non–small cell lung cancer • Surgery • VATS • Elderly • COPD • Preoperative assessment

KEY POINTS

- Newer techniques in intraoperative and postoperative management allow surgeons to successfully treat patients that were not eligible for surgery in the past.
- Evidence supports the use of minimally invasive surgery or video-assisted thoracic surgery techniques to minimize the risk of complications in marginal patients.
- Factors that affect or modify the patients' true forced expiratory volume of air in 1 second in the immediate postoperative period may be more important than the predicted postoperative physiologic parameters.
- The surgical approach needs to be a deciding factor in the treatment of marginal patients.
- Marginal patients should be seen in a multidisciplinary setting with the input of thoracic surgeons that can provide the full suite of surgical options.

INTRODUCTION

In this day and age of minimally invasive surgery (MIS), cyber knives, computed tomography (CT) screening, and increasing life expectancy (as well as increasing patient expectations), the question of defining the limits of resection in terms of pulmonary function is more germane than ever before. Classic guidelines, or cutoffs, from historical controls have been circumvented by newer techniques in intraoperative and postoperative management and have allowed surgeons to successfully treat patients who were not eligible for surgery in the past.

HISTORICAL CONTEXT

Dr King from Massachusetts General Hospital may have been one of the first surgeons to comment on what is now intuitively obvious to us: pulmonary complications are the most common cause of early postoperative morbidity and mortality.[1] He noted in his paper in 1932 that following laparotomy, a "...condition of hypoventilation apparently allows the collection of secretion in the bronchi and atelectasis and pneumonia may result."[1] Further, it was shown that abdominal operations were followed by pulmonary physiologic changes, including marked reductions in vital capacity.

From these observations made in the general surgery arena, the advent of spirometry in the 1950s enabled a relatively repeatable and quantifiable assessment of pulmonary function to be performed.[2,3] The next breakthrough in the effects of marginal lung function on patient outcomes came with Gaensler and colleagues'[3] seminal work published in 1955, which showed the value of preoperative spirometric assessment in patients undergoing surgery for

No conflicts of interest to disclose.
Department of Surgery, St Vincent's Hospital, University of Melbourne, 55 Victoria Parade, Melbourne, Victoria 3065, Australia
E-mail address: nzalam@gmail.com

Thorac Surg Clin 24 (2014) 361–369
http://dx.doi.org/10.1016/j.thorsurg.2014.07.004
1547-4127/14/$ – see front matter © 2014 Elsevier Inc. All rights reserved.

thoracic.theclinics.com

pulmonary tuberculosis.[4] In particular, FEV_1 came to predominance as a predictor of postoperative risk.

Further refinement was required, however, as pointed out by Kohman and colleagues[5] in the 1980s. In analyzing predictable risks for mortality following thoracotomy for lung cancer, they were only able to account for 12% of observed mortality, with the remaining mortality being ascribed to chance or, more likely, to previously unrecognized factors.

Enter diffusion capacity. Ferguson and colleagues[6] discovered that diffusion capacity of carbon monoxide (DLCO) was the most important predictor of mortality after pulmonary resection. This discovery led to the widespread evaluation of DLCO and not just spirometry in patients undergoing pulmonary resection.

CURRENT GUIDELINES

The current guidelines from the American College of Chest Physicians (ACCP), the British Thoracic Society (BTS), and the European Respiratory Society (ERS) are shown in **Figs. 1–3**, respectively.[7–9] These recommendations, which would be familiar to any thoracic surgeon who has practiced in the past 30 years, are based largely on 3 case series published in the 1970s with a total of more than 2000 patients. These guidelines certainly serve as the gold standard, but there have clearly been several changes in practice that are not necessarily addressed.

Previous iterations of these guidelines were less comprehensive, but the current set does acknowledge the limitations of the guideline process and offers some instructive suggestions as to when it may be possible to identify specific patient subgroups that have a differing risk profile. For example, in the BTS' guidelines, it is noted that lung volume reduction surgery (LVRS) criteria should be considered, as some patients may actually have improved lung function following resection.

However, there is some question regarding the significance of these guidelines.

WORST-CASE FORCED EXPIRATORY VOLUME IN THE FIRST SECOND OF EXPIRATION

The guidelines all rely heavily on the calculation of the predictive postoperative (ppo) values of FEV_1 and DLCO. But as noted earlier, this validation was based on retrospective data. An elegant series of studies performed by Varela and colleagues[10,11] adds another dimension to the problem. In their first study, they prospectively

examined 125 patients that underwent lobectomy and compared their $ppoFEV_1$ with actually measured FEV_1 at the bedside on postoperative days (POD) 1 through 6.[10] The hypothesis was that postoperative complications generally occur in the first few POD; therefore, a measure of the true FEV_1 at that time may be valuable. The results are shown in **Fig. 4**. True FEV_1 was lowest on POD 1 (the worst-case FEV_1), when the mean was 71% of the $ppoFEV_1$ and increased each day, though it did not meet the $ppoFEV_1$ even on POD 6. There was also an inverse correlation between the true FEV_1 and pain scores.

In a follow-up study, they hypothesized that true measured FEV_1 was a better predictor of postoperative complications than $ppoFEV_1$.[11] They prospectively followed 198 patients that underwent anatomic resections and correlated the occurrence of cardiorespiratory complications with several variables. The results are shown in **Table 1**. True FEV_1 correlated most strongly with the development of complications, whereas $ppoFEV_1$ was less important than patient age and of similar importance to pain scores on POD 1 and type of analgesia.

An interesting point is that they also examined the effect of video-assisted thoracic surgery (VATS) versus thoracotomy and found it to be relatively unimportant as a predictor of complications. This finding may be a result of several reasons. First, the study was multi-institutional and there were no VATS guidelines. Second, there are no data on how many of the cases were VATS procedures. Third, there is no description of the actual VATS techniques used (ie, whether these were true thoracoscopic procedures with no rib spreading or whether they were video-assisted operations whereby the camera acts largely as a light source and the ribs are still spread to a degree).

SPECIFIC CONSIDERATIONS

These insights suggest that the picture is not simple. Factors that affect or modify patients' true FEV_1 in the immediate postoperative period may be more important than the predicted postoperative physiologic parameters that are the foundations of the guidelines. Other studies have gone on to suggest what some of those factors may be.

MINIMALLY INVASIVE SURGERY

Nakata and colleagues[12] looked specifically at the role of MIS or VATS techniques in postoperative lung function. In a nonrandomized study they

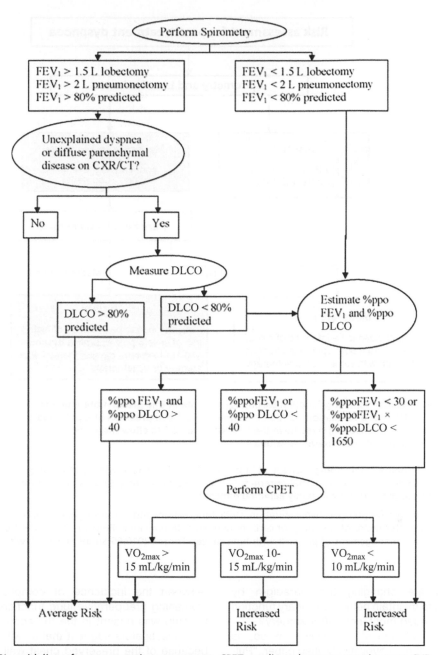

Fig. 1. ACCP's guidelines for preoperative assessment. CPET, cardio pulmonary exercise test; CXR, chest x-ray; VO_{2max}, maximum oxygen consumption. (*Adapted from* Brunelli A, Kim AW, Berger KI, et al. Physiologic evaluation of the patient with lung cancer being considered for resectional surgery. Chest 2013;143(5 Suppl):e166S–90S; with permission.)

compared 11 patients that had open lobectomy with 10 patients that had VATS lobectomy and examined their postoperative lung function.[12] It should be noted that some patients were selected for VATS if their preoperative lung function was poor. Pulmonary function was measured at POD 7, POD 14, and in the late phase (defined as approximately 1 year after surgery). As seen in

Fig. 5, the peak flows achieved on POD 7 and 14 by patients who had undergone VATS were significantly better than those who had undergone thoracotomy, with the groups converging at the 1-year mark.

This finding is compelling because we know that most complications occur in the early postoperative period. Could it be that MIS or VATS

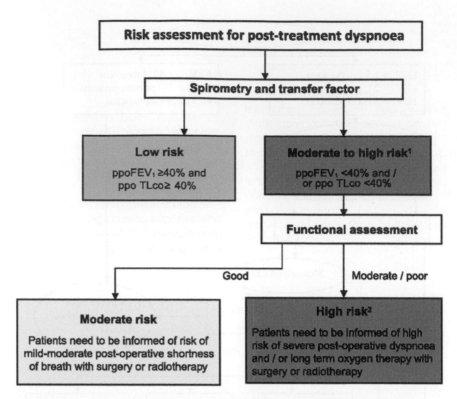

1. **Consider split lung function testing for patients in this group if there is any suspicion of a ventilation perfusion mismatch (e.g. compression of a pulmonary artery or marked emphysema in the lobe with cancer) to allow more accurate estimation of post-operative values.**

2. **Patients in this sub-group are at high risk of ventilator dependency after surgery. It is important to ensure that criteria for LVRS have been considered as lung function can improve in appropriately selected patients.**

Fig. 2. BTS' guidelines for preoperative evaluation. LVRS, lung volume reduction surgery; ppo, predictive postoperative; TLCO, transfer factor of the lung for carbon monoxide. (*From* Lim E, Baldwin D, Beckles M, et al. Guidelines on the radical management of patients with lung cancer. Thorax 2010;65(Suppl 3):iii1–27; with permission.)

techniques are changing the paradigm by enabling us to maintain better pulmonary function when it is needed most, right after surgery?

Berry and colleagues[13] certainly think so, as evidenced by their provocatively titled paper, "Pulmonary function tests do not predict pulmonary complications after thoracoscopic lobectomy."[13] They looked at 340 patients with impaired pulmonary function who underwent lobectomy. This group was defined as having preoperative DLCO or FEV_1 of less than 60% of predicted. A total of 173 patients had a thoracoscopic operation, and 167 had thoracotomy. They then correlated the incidence of pulmonary complications with the preoperative pulmonary function tests. The results are shown in **Fig. 6**.

As seen, when thoracotomy was performed, there was an effective dose-response relationship

between the incidence of complications and worsening preoperative lung function. This relationship was absent in the thoracoscopy group. The investigators suggest that an MIS approach, because of the preserved chest wall mechanics and less pain, enables them to perform surgery on patients with poorer lung function with the same risk as those patients with better preoperative lung function.

These results are from a high-volume specialist center and are most likely biased. However, data from a more generalized set of surgeons and patients corroborates these findings. Ceppa and colleagues[14] examined the Society of Thoracic Surgeons' database, a national multi-institutional dataset, and queried whether there were benefits from a VATS approach in high-risk patients. They included almost 13,000 patients (12,970, with

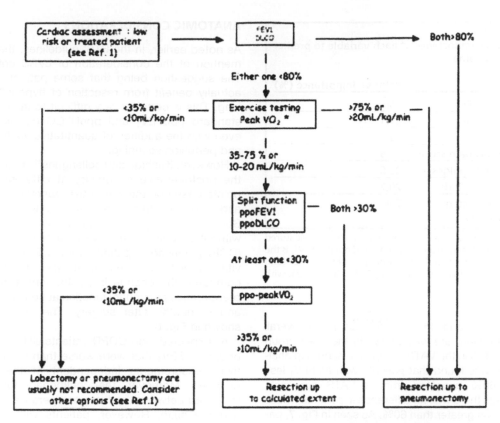

Fig. 3. ERS' guidelines for resection. CPET, cardio pulmonary exercise test; ppo, predictive postoperative; VO$_2$, oxygen consumption per minute. (*Adapted from* Bolliger CT, Perruchoud AP. Functional evaluation of the lung resection candidate. Eur Respir J 1998;11:198–212.)

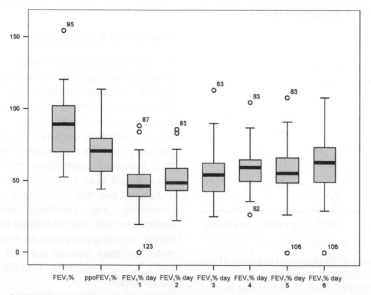

Fig. 4. Comparison of preoperative FEV$_1$, ppoFEV$_1$, and measured postoperative FEV$_1$ on POD 1 to 6. (*From* Varela G, Brunelli A, Rocco G, et al. Predicted vs observed FEV1 in the immediate postoperative period after pulmonary lobectomy. Eur J Cardiothorac Surg 2006;30(4):644–8; with permission.)

Table 1	
Relative importance of each variable to predict the outcome	
Variable	Relative Importance (%)
First-day FEV_1	100
Patient age	51.1
ppoFEV_1	43
First-day pain score	41.9
Epidural analgesia	35.6
Body mass index	29.7
Video-assisted procedure	7.4

Adapted from Varela G, Brunelli A, Rocco G, et al. Measured FEV1 in the first postoperative day, and not ppoFEV1, is the best predictor of cardio-respiratory morbidity after lung resection. Eur J Cardiothorac Surg 2007;31(3):518–21; with permission.

8439 open and 4531 VATS cases). The overall complication rate was 21.7% in the open group and 17.8% in the VATS group. In a subgroup analysis, it was found that patients with an FEV_1 less than 60% benefited from a VATS approach, whereas there was no difference in patients whose FEV_1 was greater than 60%. As seen in **Fig. 7**, patients with a lower predicted FEV_1 were better served by a VATS procedure.

There is certainly a growing body of evidence suggesting that, with MIS techniques, the morbidity and mortality of patients with marginal pulmonary function can be minimized. Hence, the surgical approach needs to be a deciding factor in the treatment of marginal patients.

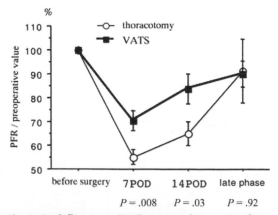

Fig. 5. Peak flow rates (PFR) expressed as a ratio of preoperative values measured after surgery (VATS vs thoracotomy). (*From* Nakata M, Saeki H, Yokoyama N, et al. Pulmonary function after lobectomy: video-assisted thoracic surgery vs thoracotomy. Ann Thorac Surg 2000;70(3):938–41; with permission.)

ANATOMIC CONSIDERATIONS

As noted earlier, in the BTS' guidelines, there is mention of the consideration of LVRS criteria. The suggestion being that some patients may actually benefit from resection of hyperinflated lung. This is certainly very difficult to factor into standard ppoFEV_1 and ppoDLCO calculations even with the addition of quantitative ventilation and perfusion scanning.

However, Kushibe and colleagues[15] measured the postoperative spirometry at different time points based on the site of the lobectomy to try and explore this interesting phenomenon. Specifically, they looked at patients with and without chronic obstructive pulmonary disease (COPD), defined as patients with an FEV_1/forced vital capacity ratio less than 70%. They then compared the change in postoperative versus preoperative pulmonary function at both 1 month and 6 months after surgery. The results are shown in **Fig. 8**.

As expected, non-COPD patients all had postoperative FEV_1 that were worse than preoperative measurements independent of the lobe resected. Moreover, their pulmonary function improved between the first postoperative month and the sixth. However, patients with COPD who had upper lobectomies actually did better than non-COPD patients when looking at their percentage change in lung function. Patients with COPD who had right upper lobectomies (RUL) actually had better pulmonary function after surgery and continued to improve at 6 months postoperatively, a true LVRS effect.

SUBLOBAR RESECTIONS

The choice of sublobar resections (preferably segmentectomy but also wedge resections) for lung cancer remains controversial. It is also a topic that is beyond the scope of this paper. However, there are some data that help support the use of these options in certain patient groups. The first priority is always a complete resection, but within that framework are there marginal groups that may benefit from sublobar resections?

At play are the competing risks of additional morbidity and mortality with a lobectomy compared with the additional risk of tumor recurrence. In marginal patients who have competing risks on their overall survival, there likely is a point when a sublobar resection may confer an advantage.

This topic was explored in a paper by Mery and colleagues.[16] They examined the Surveillance, Epidemiology, and End Results database

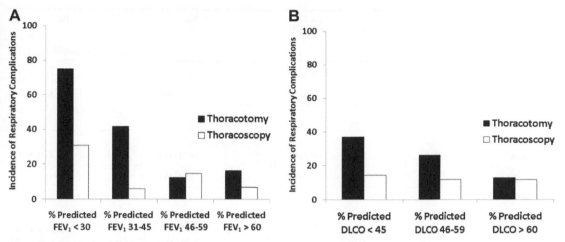

Fig. 6. Incidence of respiratory complications as function of (A) preoperative FEV_1 and (B) preoperative DLCO. (*From* Berry MF, Villamizar-Ortiz NR, Tong BC, et al. Pulmonary function tests do not predict pulmonary complications after thoracoscopic lobectomy. Ann Thorac Surg 2010;89(4):1044–51 [discussion: 1051–2]; with permission.)

to determine the effect of age and the extent of surgery on survival in lung cancer. They analyzed 14,555 patients who were initially divided into 3 age groups: those younger than 65 years, those aged 65 to 74 years, and those older than 74 years. In the final analysis (**Fig. 9**), they noted that a survival advantage for lobectomy over limited resections was present for patients aged 71 years and younger but that it disappeared for patients aged 72 years and older.

DISCUSSION

Decision making in potentially curable lung cancer is in many ways an exercise in risk-benefit analysis. Although surgery remains the gold standard for curative therapy in early stage lung cancer, the stakes are highest with marginal patients. With these patients, the standard operating metrics do not apply. First, their surgical risks are higher. Second, their expected benefits may be lower because of competing risks from

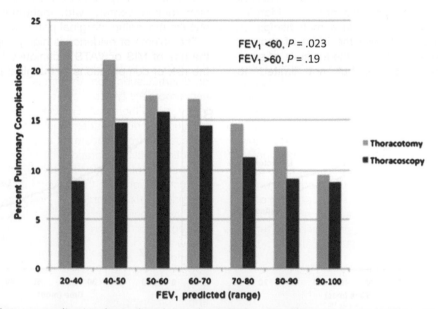

Fig. 7. Respiratory complications by predicted FEV_1, thoracotomy versus thoracoscopy. (*From* Ceppa DP, Kosinski AS, Berry MF, et al. Thoracoscopic lobectomy has increasing benefit in patients with poor pulmonary function: a Society of Thoracic Surgeons Database analysis. Ann Surg 2012;256(3):487–93; with permission.)

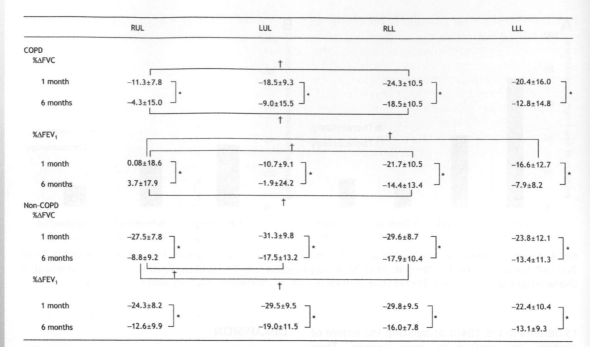

	RUL	LUL	RLL	LLL
COPD				
%ΔFVC		†		
1 month	−11.3±7.8	−18.5±9.3	−24.3±10.5	−20.4±16.0
6 months	−4.3±15.0	−9.0±15.5	−18.5±10.5	−12.8±14.8
		†		
%ΔFEV₁			†	
		†		
1 month	0.08±18.6	−10.7±9.1	−21.7±10.5	−16.6±12.7
6 months	3.7±17.9	−1.9±24.2	−14.4±13.4	−7.9±8.2
Non-COPD		†		
%ΔFVC				
1 month	−27.5±7.8	−31.3±9.8	−29.6±8.7	−23.8±12.1
6 months	−8.8±9.2	−17.5±13.2	−17.9±10.4	−13.4±11.3
		†		
%ΔFEV₁		†		
1 month	−24.3±8.2	−29.5±9.5	−29.8±9.5	−22.4±10.4
6 months	−12.6±9.9	−19.0±11.5	−16.0±7.8	−13.1±9.3

COPD, chronic obstructive pulmonary disease; RUL, right upper lobectomy; LUL, left upper lobectomy; RLL, right lower lobectomy; LLL, left lower lobectomy; %ΔFVC, percentage change in forced vital capacity; %ΔFEV₁, percentage change in forced expiratory volume in 1 s. *P<.05 1 month vs. 6 months at the same percentage change and site of lobectomy. †P<.05 RUL vs. other lobectomy at the same percentage change and evaluation time.

Fig. 8. Percentage change in preoperative and postoperative pulmonary function at early and late evaluation times, patients with COPD versus non-COPD patients. (*From* Kushibe K, Kawaguchi T, Kimura M, et al. Influence of the site of lobectomy and chronic obstructive pulmonary disease on pulmonary function: a follow-up analysis. Interact Cardiovasc Thorac Surg 2009;8(5):529–33; with permission.)

comorbidities, such as cardiac disease, COPD, or other cancers. Therefore, it behooves surgeons to be critical, not only of the available data but also of their own practice. Marginal patients should be seen in a multidisciplinary setting and should have the input of thoracic surgeons who can provide the full suite of surgical options including, but not limited to, bronchoplastic and arterioplastic reconstructions, segmentectomies, and MIS or VATS techniques. They should also be treated in high-volume centers with institutional experience in managing marginal patients.

The volume of evidence is highly supportive of the use of MIS or VATS techniques to minimize the risk of complications in marginal patients. In

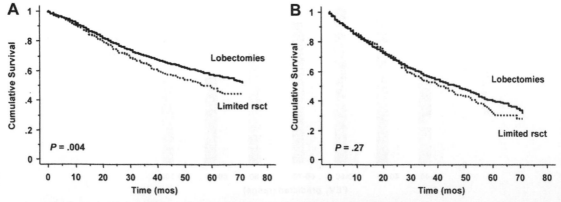

Fig. 9. Overall survival for patients ≤71 (*A*) and ≥72 (*B*). (*From* Mery CM, Pappas AN, Bueno R, et al. Similar long-term survival of elderly patients with non-small cell lung cancer treated with lobectomy or wedge resection within the surveillance, epidemiology, and end results database. Chest 2005;128:237–45; with permission.)

addition, case-by-case analysis is mandatory to enable the input of dedicated surgeons to those patients with specific anatomic situations, such as RUL tumors in patients with heterogeneous emphysema. These patients may be marginal on paper and, as such, would certainly not pass the guideline cutoffs approach. Similarly, patients with smaller tumors that can be resected with VATS segmentectomies may also be missed unless all patients with early stage disease are discussed in a team setting.

SUMMARY

The advent of MIS or VATS techniques, better perioperative anesthesia management, and better postoperative care enables thoracic surgeons to operate on marginal patients, with less risk than previously established. Careful preoperative decision making in a multidisciplinary setting should insure that all patients are given the best potential curative option.

REFERENCES

1. King DS. Postoperative pulmonary complications: a statistical study based on two years' personal observation. Surg Gynecol Obstet 1932;56:43–50.
2. Miller WF, Wu N, Johnson RL. Convenient method for evaluating pulmonary ventilatory function with a single breath test. Anesthesiology 1956;17(3): 480–93.
3. Gaensler EA, Cugell DW, Lindgren I, et al. The role of pulmonary insufficiency in mortality and invalidism following surgery for pulmonary tuberculosis. J Thorac Surg 1955;29(2):163–87.
4. Woodruff W, Merkel CG, Wright GW. Decision in thoracic surgery as influenced by the knowledge of pulmonary physiology. J Thorac Surg 1953; 26(2):156–83.
5. Kohman LJ, Meyer JA, Ikins PM, et al. Random versus predictable risks of mortality after thoracotomy for lung cancer. J Thorac Cardiovasc Surg 1986;91(4):551–4.
6. Ferguson MK, Little L, Rizzo L, et al. Diffusion capacity predicts morbidity and mortality after pulmonary

resection. J Thorac Cardiovasc Surg 1988;96(6): 894–900.
7. Brunelli A, Kim AW, Berger KI, et al. Physiologic evaluation of the patient with lung cancer being considered for resectional surgery. Chest 2013; 143(5 suppl):e166S–90S.
8. Lim E, Baldwin D, Beckles M, et al. Guidelines on the radical management of patients with lung cancer. Thorax 2010;65(Suppl 3):iii1–27.
9. Brunelli A, Charloux A, Bolliger CT, et al. ERS/ESTS clinical guidelines on fitness for radical therapy in lung cancer patients (surgery and chemo-radiotherapy). Eur Respir J 2009;34(1):17–41. http://dx.doi.org/10.1183/09031936.00184308.
10. Varela G, Brunelli A, Rocco G, et al. Predicted versus observed FEV1 in the immediate postoperative period after pulmonary lobectomy. Eur J Cardiothorac Surg 2006;30(4):644–8.
11. Varela G, Brunelli A, Rocco G, et al. Measured FEV1 in the first postoperative day, and not ppoFEV1, is the best predictor of cardio-respiratory morbidity after lung resection. Eur J Cardiothorac Surg 2007; 31(3):518–21.
12. Nakata M, Saeki H, Yokoyama N, et al. Pulmonary function after lobectomy: video-assisted thoracic surgery versus thoracotomy. Ann Thorac Surg 2000;70(3):938–41.
13. Berry MF, Villamizar-Ortiz NR, Tong BC, et al. Pulmonary function tests do not predict pulmonary complications after thoracoscopic lobectomy. Ann Thorac Surg 2010;89(4):1044–51 [discussion: 1051–2].
14. Ceppa DP, Kosinski AS, Berry MF, et al. Thoracoscopic lobectomy has increasing benefit in patients with poor pulmonary function: a Society of Thoracic Surgeons database analysis. Ann Surg 2012;256(3): 487–93.
15. Kushibe K, Kawaguchi T, Kimura M, et al. Influence of the site of lobectomy and chronic obstructive pulmonary disease on pulmonary function: a follow-up analysis. Interact Cardiovasc Thorac Surg 2009; 8(5):529–33.
16. Mery CM, Pappas AN, Bueno R, et al. Similar long-term survival of elderly patients with non-small cell lung cancer treated with lobectomy or wedge resection within the Surveillance, Epidemiology, and End Results database. Chest 2005;128:237–45.

Surgical Resection of Lung Cancer in the Elderly

Carlos Bravo-Iñiguez, MD, Mauricio Perez Martinez, MD, Katherine W. Armstrong, MPH, Michael Thomas Jaklitsch, MD*

KEYWORDS

- Elderly • Lung cancer • Resection • Functional status • Preoperative evaluation

KEY POINTS

- Assessment for thoracic surgery in elderly patients should be based on physiologic rather than chronologic age.
- The best predictor for a surgical outcome in the elderly population is functional status; therefore, an assessment to identify frailty is indispensable.
- Particular operative strategies are used to approach surgical resection in the elderly, including the use of video-assisted thoracoscopic surgery and limited resections.
- A thorough preoperative assessment is imperative to determine whether a patient is an appropriate surgical candidate, and to predict and avoid postoperative complications.

INTRODUCTION: NATURE OF THE PROBLEM

Surgical resection of lung cancer in the elderly is a common practice in today's clinical setting, but overlooking the frail patient can turn out to be deadly. Although there are different definitions of elderly, from the traditional "65 years or older" to the more commonly accepted "70 years and older," nearly all thoracic surgeons have gained experience in operating successfully within this cohort. After all, lung cancer rates are highest in the elderly. The median age of diagnosis in the United States is 70 years, and 68% of patients are diagnosed after age 65. In 2014 an estimated of 224,210 Americans will be diagnosed and 159,260 will die of lung cancer, more than 110,000 of whom will be older than 65 years.[1] There is a difference, however, between operating on carefully selected elderly patients and routinely offering surgical intervention for all patients older than 65. Surgeons need to identify frail elderly patients who will not benefit from surgical resection.

The American population is getting old. The current life expectancy within the United States is 78.7 years and increasing (compared with an average life expectancy of 49 years in 1900). By 2050 more than 20% of the population will be older than 65 years.[2,3] In general, the very elderly population is heterogeneous. We are no longer amazed by marathon runners older than 80, yet any nursing home has nonfunctional patients younger than 75 years. For this reason, age alone cannot be used as a single guide to offer or refuse surgical therapy. Furthermore, as clinicians maintain that the biology of lung cancer may also be heterogeneous in the very elderly, a wider range of therapies may be applicable to this group. The use of reliable preoperative assessments is critical in the selection of therapy for each patient. The best predictor for a surgical outcome in the elderly population is functional status; therefore, an assessment to identify frailty is indispensable. Standard preoperative assessment tools may prove less reliable in the identification of occult frail

The authors have nothing to disclose.
Division of Thoracic Surgery, Brigham and Women's Hospital, Harvard Medical School, 75 Francis Street, Boston, MA 02115, USA
* Corresponding author.
E-mail address: mjaklitsch@partners.org

Thorac Surg Clin 24 (2014) 371–381
http://dx.doi.org/10.1016/j.thorsurg.2014.07.001

patients who are hiding their disability from providers, family members, and themselves. The authors advocate and, furthermore, discuss in this article the routine use of new assessment tools to identify this population and to better tailor individual therapies.

Surgical resection for non–small cell lung cancer (NSCLC) offers the best chance for cure if the disease is detected in the early stages. Early-stage disease is more commonly encountered with increasing age at presentation. The authors' analysis of a cohort of 14,555 patients with early-stage NSCLC in the Surveillance, Epidemiology, and End Results (SEER) database in 2005 showed that the frequency of stage I disease increased from 79% in patients younger than 65 to 87% in patients age 75 or older.[4] Other investigators have also noted an increase in surgically resectable disease as a function of increasing age. In the Centralized Cancer Patient Data System database of 22,874 patients with lung cancer of all stages, O'Rourke and colleagues[5] found that 15.3% of those aged 54 years or younger had surgically resectable disease, whereas 25% of those aged 74 years or older had resectable disease.

Elderly patients also have a more frequent incidence of squamous cell carcinoma (SCC), a histology that is more likely associated with local disease and lower recurrence, and may have longer survival times.[6–8] Analysis of the SEER database showed that the frequency of SCC increased from 27% in patients younger than 65 years to 38% in patients 75 years and older, with parallel decreases in frequency of adenocarcinoma from 61% to 50% in corresponding age groups, as depicted in **Fig. 1**.[4] It is not unusual to encounter a large peripheral SCC with no nodal metastases in the elderly patient.

THERAPEUTIC OPTIONS AND/OR SURGICAL TECHNIQUES

Lobectomy, removal of 1 of the 5 lobes of the lung and associated lymph nodes within a single pleural membrane, is considered the standard of care for surgical resection of early-stage NSCLC.[9] A limited resection is an alternative in the elderly, high-risk population because of the ability to spare functional lung tissue. In a study conducted by Mery and colleagues[4] at the Brigham and Women's Hospital using data from SEER from 1992 to 1997, investigators calculated that lobectomies and limited resections have similar overall survival for the first 25 months, but differ after 25 months in patients younger than 71 years. Survival benefits of lobectomies were not observed for patients older than 71, making the lung-sparing alternative a more attractive option for this age group.

Particular operative strategies are used to approach surgical resection in the elderly, including

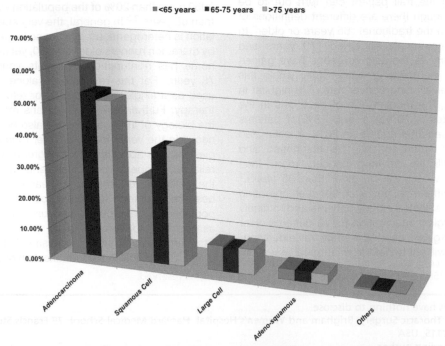

Fig. 1. Lung cancer histology by age. (*Data from* Mery CM, Pappas AN, Bueno R, et al. Similar long-term survival of elderly patients with non-small cell lung cancer treated with lobectomy or wedge resection within the Surveillance, Epidemiology, and End Results database. Chest 2005;128:237–45.)

the use of video-assisted thoracoscopic surgery (VATS) to minimize chest wall trauma and by consideration of limited resections for the most elderly to minimize loss of lung tissue. VATS is a minimally invasive surgery performed through 2 or 3 incisions of 2 cm in length. A utility incision less than 6 to 8 cm long may be used, without spreading of the ribs. VATS procedures in the elderly have been shown to have lower morbidity and lower rates of postoperative delirium, and result in earlier ambulation, a lower narcotic requirement, and a faster recovery time.[10–14] As early as 1996 the authors reported their initial experience with 307 cases, demonstrating that minimally invasive procedures can be performed safely with low morbidity and mortality in high-risk elderly patients. There is a natural decay of pulmonary function in the elderly owing to the following factors: respiratory muscle atrophy, reduction in force-generating capacity of residual muscle, ossification of costal cartilage, and changed mechanics of breathing. Making an open thoracotomy causes disruption of the mechanics of breathing and places the elderly patient at particular risk for postoperative pneumonia.

Multiple studies emphasize the undertreatment of cancer in the elderly.[15] Published data from the SEER database showed that approximately 30% of the most elderly patients In the database were denied surgery or were offered only palliative surgery, in contrast to only 8% of the youngest patients.[4] Many clinicians consider not offering surgery to octogenarians, based on the premise that their natural life expectancy is less than the rate of growth of their suspected lung cancer. This axiom is frequently not true.

Using 2009 data, the life expectancy of an 80-year-old in the United States is 9.1 years (8.2 years for men, 9.7 years for women), whereas the median survival for elderly patients with untreated early-stage lung cancer is only 14 months.[16] These data suggest that life limitation for an 80-year-old person with lung cancer is likely to be cancer related.[17]

Table 1[18] shows life table data from 2009 for patients older than 65 years.

CLINICAL OUTCOMES AND THE PREOPERATIVE ASSESSMENT
Physiologic Changes of Age

Physiologic changes of the respiratory system associated with aging include reduced chest wall compliance with stiffening of calcified costal cartilages, diminished diaphragmatic excursion, and narrowing of the intervertebral disk space. There is a reduction of lung elastic recoil with loss of alveolar architecture, producing decreased surface

Table 1			
Life expectancy by age, United States, 2009			
Age (y)	**Total**[a]	**Male**[a]	**Female**[a]
65	19.1	17.6	20.3
70	15.5	14.2	16.5
75	12.1	11	12.9
80	9.1	8.2	9.7
85	6.6	5.9	7
90	4.7	4.1	4.9

[a] Additional years of life.

Adapted from Arias E. United States life tables, 2009. National vital statistics reports; vol 62 no 7. Hyattsville, MD: National Center for Health Statistics. 2014.

alveolar gas exchange. Progressive atrophy creates weakness of the respiratory musculature. In addition, there is a decrease in central nervous system responsiveness. The loss of lung elastic recoil and decreased lung compliance diminishes negative intrapleural pressure, which then prevents reopening of the small airways, resulting in air trapping and inadequate ventilation. Functionally this manifests in a gradual decline of vital capacity and partial pressure of oxygen, with an increased residual volume. Decline in motor power of the accessory muscles and a stiffening of the chest wall also result in a declining forced expiratory volume in 1 second (FEV_1). Changes in lung compliance are not uniformly distributed. Higher respiratory rates therefore increase ventilation-perfusion mismatch. The elderly also exhibit a blunted ventilatory response to both hypoxic and hypercapnic insults.[19,20] Physiologic changes in lung mechanics make elderly patients particularly sensitive to narcotics and muscle relaxants, and to supine positioning. In addition, elderly patients are at increased risk for respiratory tract infections, owing to waning immune responses.[21] Smoking in particular has been shown to cause bronchial mucociliary dysfunction,[22] which has been associated with increased susceptibility to infection.[23]

Increasing age is also associated with declines in other organ systems. There is a decline in glomerular filtration rate, an increasing incidence of heart disease, and an increasing incidence of cognitive dysfunction. Changes in body composition decrease the volume of distribution of water-soluble drugs.[24] In addition, elderly patients take more medications in comparison with younger patients, and are vulnerable to adverse drug effects.

Preoperative Evaluation

Elderly patients are at increased risk for postoperative morbidity and mortality because of comorbid conditions and a decreased ability to recover physiologic homeostasis after surgical stress. Older patients represent a heterogeneous population, and should be offered surgery on the basis of physiologic rather than chronologic age. A thorough preoperative assessment is imperative to determine whether a patient is an appropriate surgical candidate and to predict and avoid postoperative complications. Geriatric assessment tools that specifically assess patients' functional status, aimed at predicting outcomes in the elderly surgical population, remain under study.

Cardiac Risk Assessment

The American Heart Association (AHA) and American College of Cardiology (ACC) published a readily accessible consensus practice guideline on perioperative cardiovascular evaluation for noncardiac surgery that provides a template for assessing patients of all ages.[25] The AHA/ACC guidelines describe a stepwise approach to preoperative surgery with risk stratification and further imaging, determined by evaluating symptoms, clinical predictors, and functional capacity. Six independent predictors of complications were identified in the guideline modifications by Auerbach and Goldman[26] in 2006, and were included in the Revised Cardiac Risk Index (RCRI)[27]: high-risk surgery, history of ischemic heart disease, history of congestive heart failure, history of cerebrovascular disease, preoperative treatment with insulin, and preoperative creatinine level of greater than 2.0 mg/dL. Rates of major cardiac complications with 0, 1, 2, or 3 or more criteria were 0.5%, 1.3%, 4%, and 9%, respectively. Thoracic surgery was defined as high risk.

Clinical history should focus on assessment for coronary risk factors and physical capacity, including the ability to climb 2 flights of stairs or walk 1 block. In general, patients with poor functional status, 1 to 2 RCRI criteria, or with a history of angina or claudication should undergo noninvasive testing. An electrocardiogram (ECG) should be performed in every patient undergoing a thoracic procedure. If the ECG shows an abnormality or if it is difficult to determine whether the pathologic cause of symptoms is cardiac or pulmonary, there should be a low threshold for additional cardiac imaging and an assessment by a cardiologist to assist in risk stratification.

Adrenergic modification with β-blockers in the perioperative period for patients undergoing thoracic surgery serves to both reduce the risk of myocardial infarction (MI) and prevent postoperative supraventricular tachycardias. The RCRI criteria have also been used to determine the need for perioperative β-blocker and statin therapy to prevent MI or other cardiac complications. Patients with 2 or more RCRI criteria (thoracic surgery patients undergoing a resection by definition have at least 1 criterion) and no long-term indication for β-blockade should receive β-blockers at the time of surgery and optimally continue them for 1 month, or indefinitely if they have appropriate medical histories such as prior MI.[28]

Pulmonary Risk Assessment

All patients undergoing lung resection surgery should have pulmonary function tests performed. FEV_1 by spirometry is the most common measured value used to determine a patient's suitability for surgery. Data obtained in the 1970s from more than 2000 patients showed a mortality rate of less than 5% for patients with an FEV_1 greater than 1.5 L for lobectomy and greater than 2 L for pneumonectomy.[29] In reviewing more recent spirometry studies performed from 1994 to 2000, Datta and Lahiri[30] concluded that in NSCLC patients, increased postoperative morbidity and mortality were predicted by an FEV_1 of less than 2 L or less than 60% predicted for pneumonectomy, and FEV_1 of less than 1.6 L for lobectomy and less than 0.6 L for wedge or segmentectomy.[30]

Lung resections have of course been undertaken in patients with much poorer lung function. In 2005 Linden and colleagues[31] published data from a series of 100 consecutive patients with preoperative FEV_1 of less than 35% predicted undergoing lung tumor resection. In this series there was a 1% mortality rate and a 36% complication rate. Eleven patients were discharged with a new oxygen requirement, 4 patients developed pneumonia, 1 patient became ventilator dependent, and 3 patients required intubation for longer than 48 hours. Twenty-two percent of patients had prolonged air leaks.

Ferguson and colleagues[32] found preoperative diffusion capacity for carbon monoxide (DLCO) to be more predictive of postoperative mortality than FEV_1 in a study of 237 patients. In this study, a DLCO of less than 60% predicted was associated with increased mortality and a DLCO of less than 80% predicted was predictive of increased pulmonary complications. Other studies, however, have not found DLCO to be a significant predictor of postoperative complications.[33,34] DLCO and spirometry may be used as complementary tests, particularly in patients with diffuse parenchymal disease or dyspnea that is out of proportion to the FEV_1, with a low DLCO prompting further evaluation.[35]

Formal and simple exercise testing evaluates the cardiopulmonary system under induced physiologic stress, and also has been found to be predictive of postoperative complications. Girish and colleagues[28] prospectively studied symptom-limited stair climbing in patients undergoing thoracic and upper abdominal surgery. No complications occurred in patients who could climb 7 flights of stairs, whereas 89% of patients unable to climb 1 flight of stairs had complications. Inability to climb 2 flights of stairs had a positive predictive value of 80%. The ability of patients to climb stairs was found to be inversely related to the length of postoperative hospital stay.

The 6-minute walk test (6MWT) measures the distance walked over a period of 6 minutes. In a qualitative review, Solway and colleagues[36] concluded that the 6MWT was easy to administer and was more reflective of activities of daily living than other walk tests. Although stair climbing and the 6MWT are easy to perform, their use in elderly patients may be limited by orthopedic impairments, peripheral vascular insufficiency, or neurologic impairments.

As published previously,[37] a recommended preoperative pulmonary evaluation for an elderly patient should consist of spirometry, DLCO, room air arterial blood gas (ABG) analysis, and exercise tolerance tests including stair climbing and 6MWT. Patients with an FEV_1 greater than 1 L and no major abnormality of other tests (FEV_1/forced vital capacity [FVC] >50%, DLCO >50% predicted, ABG partial pressure of arterial oxygen >45 mm Hg, tolerance of exercise tests) may safely proceed with surgery, including pneumonectomy (**Fig. 2**).[38]

Further evaluation for patients who fall outside these criteria include measurement of maximal oxygen consumption (Vo_2 max) testing and ventilation/perfusion scans to calculate predicted postoperative (PPO) lung function. Vo_2 max measured by formal cardiopulmonary exercise testing is helpful to further risk-stratify patients with borderline lung function. A Vo_2 max of less than 10 mL/kg/min had a very high operative morbidity (26% total in combined data) in several small case series. Vo_2 max values of 10 to 15 mL/kg/min had an intermediate perioperative morbidity (8.3% total), whereas patients with greater than 15 mg/kg/min can proceed with lung resection surgery with an acceptable mortality rate.[35]

PPO lung function can be calculated by several methods such as anatomic estimation, ventilation or perfusion scans, or quantitative computed tomography scans. PPO FEV_1 by anatomic estimation is calculated with the following formula:

$$PPO\ FEV_1 = preoperative\ FEV_1 \times (1 - \text{no. of functional or unobstructed lung segments to be removed/total no. of functional segments})$$

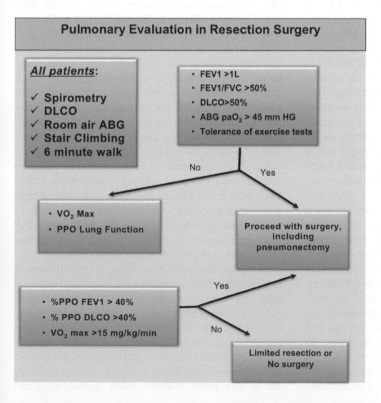

Fig. 2. Recommended pulmonary evaluation for patients undergoing lung resection. ABG, arterial blood gas; DLCO, diffusion capacity for carbon monoxide; FEV1, forced expiratory volume in 1 second; FVC, forced vital capacity; PPO, predicted postoperative; Vo2 Max, maximal oxygen consumption. (*Adapted from* Jaklitsch MT, Billmeier SE. Preoperative evaluation and risk assessment for elderly surgery patients. Thorac Surg Clin 2009;19(3):308; with permission.)

For example, in a patient with a preoperative FEV_1 of 1.5 L without previous lung resection surgery undergoing a right upper lobectomy, the PPO FEV_1 would be calculated as 1.5 L × (1 − 3/18) = 1.25 L. In a patient with a previous left lower lobectomy with an FEV_1 of 1.5 L undergoing a right lower lobectomy, the PPO FEV_1 would be 1.5 L × (1 − 5/14) = 0.96 L.

Using radionucleotide perfusion scanning, the postoperative FEV_1 is calculated by:

Postoperative FEV_1 = preoperative FEV_1 × % of radioactivity contributed by nonoperated lung

A PPO FEV_1 threshold of 0.8 L[39] or 0.7 L[40] has been suggested as a lower limit value for proceeding with lung resection. Absolute values of PPO FEV_1 can underestimate postoperative lung in people with small stature or the elderly, and can thus be converted into percent-PPO (%PPO) lung function. Multiple studies have suggested that morbidity increases at a threshold %PPO FEV_1 of less than 40%, or a %PPO DLCO of less than 40%.[32,35,41–43]

Cognitive Assessment

One of the most important pieces of information for an elderly patient is the likelihood of returning to baseline physical and mental function after surgery. Patients and their families accept that there will be a postoperative recovery time in the hospital or rehabilitation setting, but it is difficult to assess the magnitude of this functional decline and predict the risk of permanent loss of independence. There is a paucity of data assessing changes in quality of life after thoracic surgery in the elderly, and few studies that assess whether surgery triggers a postoperative loss of independence and a change in need for assistance or living requirements. A study of 68 octogenarians undergoing pulmonary resections at Johns Hopkins Medical Institutions showed that 80% of patients were discharged directly home from the hospital rather than to rehabilitation, offering some proxy information regarding immediate postoperative return to function.[44] In 1998 Moller and colleagues[45] reported a 25% rate of cognitive dysfunction at 1 week after major noncardiac surgery in elderly patients (average age 68 years), with continued dysfunction in 9% at 3 months. Data from many studies verify a high incidence of postoperative cognitive dysfunction in the first week after surgery, and dysfunction does tend to increase with age. Only one other study has substantiated long-term declines in comparison with controls, and some have suggested that declines

found in these studies may be due to random variation.[46,47] Kaneko and colleagues[48] determined that preoperative dementia was a risk factor for postoperative delirium. Furthermore, Fukuse and colleagues[49] found that thoracic surgery patients with preoperative dementia, as estimated by the Mini-Mental Status Examination (MMS), were 4-fold more likely to have postoperative complications.

Geriatric Assessments

Several assessment indices have been applied to elderly patients to determine their risk for poor outcomes. Two assessment tools specifically aimed at oncogeriatric patients are under current study and are described here.

Preoperative Assessment of Cancer in Elderly (PACE) is a tool designed by the International Society of Geriatric Oncology to assess the functional activities of oncogeriatric patients, with the goal of assessing the individualized surgical risk of these patients based on preoperative variables. Instruments used in PACE assessment include MMS, Satariano's modified index of comorbidities, activities of daily living (ADL), instrumental activities of daily living (IADL), Geriatric Depression Scale (GDS), Brief Fatigue Inventory (BFI), Eastern Cooperative Oncology Group (ECOG) performance status, American Society of Anesthesiologists score (ASA), Physiologic and Operative Severity Score for the enUmeration of Mortality and Morbidity (POSSUM), and Portsmouth (P)-POSSUM. Preliminary data analyzing PACE components has been published, assessing 30-day morbidity rates in 215 patients with a median age of 76 years who underwent surgery for breast cancer (142 patients), urogenital cancer, colorectal cancer, gastroesophageal cancer, head and neck cancer, and gynecologic cancers. In their interim results, 2 components of PACE were associated with 30-day morbidity. Lower performance status and a lower ADL score were both associated with postoperative complications. The assessment instruments MMS, GDS, BFI, and ASA were not related to 30-day morbidity.[50] Further study with a larger sample size is ongoing.

The preliminary PACE results are consistent with prior studies that correlate preoperative functional and performance status with postoperative morbidity. Functional status describes the ability to perform self-care, self-maintenance, and physical activities. Traditional measures used to assess functional status are ADL and IADL. ADL are 6 basic self-care skills, including the ability to bathe, dress, go to the toilet, transfer from a bed to chair, maintain continence, and feed oneself. IADL include higher functioning skills that are used to maintain independence in the community. This scale assesses ability to use the telephone, go shopping, prepare food, perform housekeeping and laundry, use various modes of transportation, assume responsibility for medications, and the ability to handle finances. The need for assistance in these tasks has been predictive of prolonged hospital stay, nursing home placement, and home care requirements.[51,52] Poor nutritional status, defined as a body mass index of less than 22 kg/m^2, has been associated with an increased need for assistance with ADL and a decreased 1-year survival.[53]

Performance status is a standardized scale designed to measure the ability of a patient with cancer to perform ordinary tasks. There are two scales, the Karnofsky performance scale, which ranges from 0 (dead) to 100 (normal), and the ECOG scale, ranging from 0 (asymptomatic) to 5 (dead). Comparisons of the two scales have been validated with a large sample of patients.[54] Performance status has been used to select patients for entry into chemotherapy trials; however, it is also well accepted to be associated with postoperative morbidity.[55–57]

Complications and Concerns

Mery and Jaklitsch[58] determined the 30-day postoperative mortality rate of 14,555 patients who had undergone curative resections for treating stage I or II NSCLC over the period 1992 to 1997. In an analysis of patients undergoing all types of surgery, there was a 0.45% mortality rate for those younger than 65 years, 0.6% for ages 65 to 74, and 1.2% for patients aged 75 or older ($P = .001$). Mortality differences were found to be primarily due to differences in survival of patients undergoing lobectomy, with 0.3%, 0.5%, and 1.5% mortality, respectively, for these corresponding age groups ($P = .0001$). The difference in perioperative mortality was statistically similar for patients undergoing limited resection. Prior published reports likewise did not identify a difference in expected operative mortality after thoracotomy if lung-sparing operations were performed.[59–61]

The American College of Surgeons Oncology Group (ACOSOG) Z0030 Study published morbidity and mortality data in 2006 for 1023 clinically resectable T1 or T2, N0 or nonhilar N1 NSCLC patients randomized over a period from 1999 to 2004 to undergo lymph node sampling versus mediastinal lymph node dissection. Their age-stratified morbidity and mortality data are shown in **Table 2**.[38] Of note, overall mortality was 1.4%, improved from Ginsberg's reported 3.8%, and was not statistically associated with age.[62] Ninety percent of patients in the ACOSOG Z0030 study underwent resection via a thoracotomy, with the remaining procedures performed as VATS or VATS-assisted resections. Operative mortality reported by Ginsberg for pneumonectomy and lobectomy was 6.2% and 2.9%, respectively, compared with 0% and 1.3%, in the ACOSOG study. Of note, the pneumonectomy

---

Table 2
ACOSOG Z0030 study age stratified morbidity and mortality after resection for clinically resectable T1 or T2, N0 or nonhilar N1 NSCLC

Event	Age (y)				
	<50 (n = 35)	50–59 (n = 171)	60–69 (n = 386)	70–79 (n = 361)	80+ (n = 70)
One or more complications	8 (23%)	50 (29%)	136 (35%)	162 (45%)	34 (49%)
Air leak >7 d	1 (3%)	14 (8%)	24 (6%)	33 (9%)	6 (9%)
Chest tube drainage >7 d	0	14 (8%)	42 (11%)	53 (15%)	9 (13%)
Chylothorax	1 (3%)	3 (2%)	3 (1%)	5 (1%)	1 (1%)
Hemorrhage	1 (3%)	3 (2%)	10 (3%)	16 (4%)	4 (6%)
Recurrent nerve injury	0	0	5 (1%)	2 (<1%)	0
Atrial arrhythmia	1 (3%)	13 (8%)	53 (14%)	68 (19%)	12 (17%)
Respiratory	4 (12%)	8 (5%)	30 (8%)	29 (8%)	3 (4%)
Death	1 (2.6%)	0	3 (0.8%)	8 (2.2%)	2 (2.9%)

Adapted from Jaklitsch MT, Billmeier SE. Preoperative evaluation and risk assessment for elderly surgery patients. Thorac Surg Clin 2009;19(3):304; with permission.

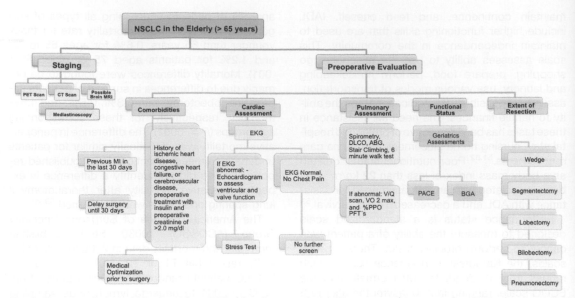

Fig. 3. Preoperative workup algorithm. BGA, blood gas analysis; CT, computed tomography; EKG, electrocardiogram; MI, myocardial infarction; MRI, magnetic resonance imaging; NSCLC, non–small cell lung cancer; PACE, Preoperative Assessment of Cancer in Elderly; PET, positron emission tomography; V/Q, ventilation/perfusion; yo, years old.

rate of the earlier study was 25.6%, versus 4% in ACOSOG, likely partially explaining the higher mortality rate of the earlier study.

The operative risk of death after pulmonary resections is largely attributable to 2 anatomic disruptions: first, the loss of functional lung tissue, and second, the morbidity and mortality introduced by the access thoracotomy.

Practical Recommendations

The authors wish to synthesize the aforementioned data into a practical plan for selecting appropriate elderly patients for surgery. The first step is to assess the stage of the disease and, thus, the amount of lung tissue that needs to be resected (**Fig. 3**). The next step is to judge operative

risk based on comorbid disease, cardiac and pulmonary function, overall functional status, and extent of surgery.

Operative risk is a probability function that depends primarily on the amount of lung resection and results of testing. **Table 3** summarizes the authors' recommendations based on years of experience caring for very elderly and frail patients. No individual item is an absolute contraindication, but provides useful parameters for a novice clinician in approaching preoperative risk assessment. All elderly patients considering thoracic surgery should have pulmonary function tests with FVC and DLCO. All should have a 6MWT, stair climbing assessment, and an estimate of Karnofsky performance status. A rare patient benefits from $Vo_{2\ max}$. This table is

Table 3
Surgical resection of lung cancer in the elderly

	Lobectomy	Lesser Resection (Segment/Wedge)	Nonoperative Therapy
Spirometry (FVC% or DLCO %PPO)	>50% PPO	25%–50% PPO	<25% PPO
6-MWT (m)	400	60–400	<60 or wheelchair
Stair climbing (no. of flights)	2	<1	Unable to climb
$Vo_{2\ max}$ (mL/kg/min)	>12	10–12	<10
Karnofsky (performance status)	70–100	30–60	<30

Abbreviations: 6-MWT, 6-minute walk test; % PPO, predicted postoperative; DLCO, diffusion capacity for carbon monoxide; FVC, forced vital capacity; $Vo_{2\ max}$, peak oxygen consumption.

intended to identify an occult frail patient, and may lead to prehabilitation before surgery or a change in the operative plan.

SUMMARY

Assessment for thoracic surgery in elderly patients should be based on physiologic rather than chronologic age. Thoracic surgery has been shown to be safe in selected elderly patients, and age should not be a contraindication to a therapy that offers the best chance of cure for patients with early-stage cancer. A targeted preoperative assessment can help individualize the risk of morbidity and mortality for each patient, and thus provide both surgeon and patient with the information needed for operative decision making. Operative interventions in the elderly require coordinated attention to the specific requirements of the aged. Specialized multidisciplinary care provided by primary care physicians, geriatric specialists, cardiologists, oncologists, surgeons, anesthetists, nurses, physical therapists, and nutrition specialists optimizes care for the elderly patient undergoing thoracic surgery. Careful selection of patients for surgery has contributed to the improvement in operative mortality over time, and refinements in preoperative testing should continue this trend in the future. The goal is to provide surgery to the maximum number of patients at the minimal cost of mortality and loss of independence.

REFERENCES

1. Howlader N, Noone AM, Krapcho M, et al. SEER cancer statistics review, 1975-2011. Bethesda (MD): National Cancer Institute; 2014. Based on November 2013 SEER data submission, posted to the SEER web site. Available at: http://seer.cancer.gov/csr/1975_2011/.
2. Kung HC, Hoyery DL, Xu J. Deaths: final data for 2005. Centers for Disease Control. Natl Vital Stat Rep 2008;56(10):1–124.
3. Vincent GK, Velkoff VA, 2010, THE NEXT FOUR DECADES, The Older Population in the United States: 2010 to 2050, Current Population Reports, P25-1138, U.S. Census Bureau, Washington, DC.
4. Mery CM, Pappas AN, Bueno R, et al. Similar long-term survival of elderly patients with non-small cell lung cancer treated with lobectomy or wedge resection within the Surveillance, Epidemiology, and End Results database. Chest 2005; 128:237–45.
5. O'Rourke MA, Feussner JR, Feigl P, et al. Age trends of lung cancer stage at diagnosis: implications for lung cancer screening in the elderly. JAMA 1987; 258:921–6.
6. Teeter SM, Holmes FF, McFarlane MJ. Lung carcinoma in the elderly population: influence of histology on the inverse relationship of stage to age. Cancer 1987;60:1331–6.
7. Weinmann M, Jeremie B, Toomes H, et al. Treatment of lung cancer in the elderly. Part I. Non-small cell lung cancer. Lung Cancer 2003;39:233–53.
8. Morandi U, Stefani A, Golinelli M, et al. Results of surgical resection in patients over the age of 70 years with non small-cell lung cancer. Eur J Cardiothorac Surg 1997;11:432–9.
9. Faulkner SL. Is Lobectomy the "gold standard" for stage I lung cancer in year 2000? Chest 2000; 118(suppl):119S.
10. Decamp MM Jr, Jaklitsch MT, Mentzer SJ, et al. The safety and versatility of video-thoracoscopy: a prospective analysis of 895 cases. J Am Coll Surg 1995;181:113–20.
11. McKenna R. Thoracoscopic lobectomy with mediastinal sampling in 80 year-old patients. Chest 1994;106:1902–4.
12. Landreneau RL, Sugarbaker DJ, Mack MJ, et al. Postoperative pain-related morbidity: video-assisted thoracic surgery versus thoracotomy. Ann Thorac Surg 1993;56:1285–9.
13. Jaklitsch MT, Bueno R, Swanson SJ, et al. Video-assisted thoracic surgery in the elderly: a review of 307 cases. Chest 1996;110:751–8.
14. Cattaneo SM, Park BJ, Wilton AS, et al. Use of video-assisted thoracic surgery for lobectomy in the elderly results in fewer complications. Ann Thorac Surg 2008;85:231–6.
15. Samet J, Hunt WC, Key C, et al. Choice of cancer therapy varies with age of patient. JAMA 1986; 255:3385–90.
16. McGarry RC, Song G, des Rosiers P, et al. Observation-only management of early stage, medically inoperable lung cancer: poor outcome. Chest 2002;121:1155–8.
17. Yellin A, Brenfield JR. Surgery for bronchogenic carcinoma in the elderly. Am Rev Respir Dis 1985;131:197.
18. Arias E. United States life tables, 2009. Natl Vital Stat Rep 2014;62(7):1–63.
19. Rossi A, Ganassini A, Tantucci C, et al. Aging and the respiratory system. Aging (Milano) 1996;8(3):143–61.
20. Janssens JP, Pache JC, Nicod LP. Physiological changes in respiratory function associated with ageing. Eur Respir J 1999;13:197–205.
21. Meyer KC. Lung infections and aging. Ageing Res Rev 2004;3(1):55–67.
22. Verra F, Escudier E, Lebargy F, et al. Ciliary abnormalities in bronchial epithelium of smokers, ex-smokers, and nonsmokers. Am J Respir Crit Care Med 1995;151(3):630–4.
23. Salathe M, O'Riordan TG, Wanner A. Treatment of mucociliary dysfunction. Chest 1996;110:1048–57.

24. McLesky CH. Anesthesia for the geriatric patient. In: Barash PG, Cullen BF, Staelting RK, editors. Clinical anesthesia. 2nd edition. Philadelphia: JB Lippincott; 1992. p. 1353–83.

25. Eagle KA, Berger PB, Calkins H, et al. ACC/AHA guideline update for perioperative cardiovascular evaluation for noncardiac surgery. Circulation 2002;105:1257–67.

26. Auerbach A, Goldman L. Assessing and reducing the cardiac risk of noncardiac surgery. Circulation 2006;113(10):1361–76.

27. Lee TH, Marcantonio MD, Mangione CM, et al. Derivation and prospective validation of a simple index for prediction of cardiac risk of major noncardiac surgery. Circulation 1999;100:1043–9.

28. Girish M, Trayner E, Dammann O, et al. Symptom-limited stair climbing as a predictor of postoperative cardiopulmonary complications after high risk surgery. Chest 2001;120:1147–51.

29. British Thoracic Society, Society of Cardiothoracic Surgeons of Great Britain and Ireland Working Party. Guidelines on the selection of patients with lung cancer for surgery. Thorax 2001;56: 89–108.

30. Datta D, Lahiri B. Preoperative evaluation of patients undergoing lung resection surgery. Chest 2003;123:2096–103.

31. Linden PA, Bueno R, Colson YL, et al. Lung resection in patients with preoperative FEV1 < 35% predicted. Chest 2005;127:1984–90.

32. Ferguson MK, Little L, Rizzo L, et al. Diffusing capacity predicts morbidity and mortality after pulmonary resection. J Thorac Cardiovasc Surg 1988;96: 894–900.

33. Stephan F, Boucheseiche S, Hollande J, et al. Pulmonary complications following lung resection: a comprehensive analysis of incidence and possible risk factors. Chest 2000;118:1263–70.

34. Botsen PC, Block AJ, Moulder PC. Relationship between preoperative pulmonary function tests and complications after thoracotomy. Surg Gynecol Obstet 1981;52:813–5.

35. Bolliger CT, Wyser C, Boser H, et al. Lung scanning and exercise testing for the prediction of postoperative performance in lung resection candidates at increased risk of complications. Chest 1995;108: 341–8.

36. Solway S, Brooks D, Lacasses Y, et al. A qualitative systematic overview of the measurement properties of functional walk tests used in the cardiorespiratory domain. Chest 2001;119(1):256–70.

37. Jaklitsch MT, Mery CM, Audisio RA. The use of surgery to treat lung cancer in elderly patients. Lancet Oncol 2003;4:463–71.

38. Jaklitsch MT, Billmeier SE. Preoperative evaluation and risk assessment for elderly surgery patients. Thorac Surg Clin 2009;19(3):301–12.

39. Olsen GN, Block AJ, Tobias JA. Prediction of postpneumonectomy pulmonary function using quantitative macroaggregate lung scanning. Chest 1974; 66:13–6.

40. Pate P, Tenholder MF, Griffin JP, et al. Preoperative assessment of the high-risk patient for lung resection. Ann Thorac Surg 1996;61:1494–500.

41. Markos J, Mullan BP, Hillman DR, et al. Preoperative assessment as a predictor of mortality and morbidity after lung resection. Am Rev Respir Dis 1989;139:902–10.

42. Holden DA, Rice TW, Stefmach K, et al. Exercise testing, 6-min walk, and stair climb in the evaluation of patients at high risk for pulmonary resection. Chest 1992;102:1774–9.

43. Wahi R, McMurtry MJ, DeCaro LF, et al. Determinants of perioperative morbidity and mortality after pneumonectomy. Ann Thorac Surg 1989;48:33–7.

44. Brock MV, Kim MP, Hooker CM, et al. Pulmonary resection in octogenarians with stage I nonsmall cell lung cancer: a 22-year experience. Ann Thorac Surg 2004;77:271–7.

45. Moller JT, Cluitmans P, Rasmussen LS, et al. Long-term postoperative cognitive dysfunction in the elderly: ISPOCD1 study. Lancet 1998;351:857–61.

46. Rasmussen LS, Siersma VD. ISPOCD group: postoperative cognitive dysfunction: true deterioration versus random variation. Acta Anaesthesiol Scand 2004;48:1137–43.

47. Newman S, Stygall J, Shaefi S, et al. Postoperative cognitive dysfunction after noncardiac surgery. Anesthesiology 2007;106:572–90.

48. Kaneko T, Takahashi S, Naka T, et al. Postoperative delirium following gastrointestinal surgery in elderly patients. Surg Today 1997;27:107–11.

49. Fukuse T, Satoda N, Hijiya K, et al. Importance of a comprehensive geriatric assessment in prediction of complications following thoracic surgery in elderly patients. Chest 2005;127:886–91.

50. Audisio RA, Ramesh H, Longo W, et al. Preoperative assessment of surgical risk in oncogeriatric patients. Oncologist 2005;10:262–8.

51. Narian O, Rubenstein L, Wieland GD, et al. Predictors of immediate and 6 month outcomes in hospitalized elderly patients. The importance of functional status. J Am Geriatr Soc 1988;36:775–83.

52. Reuben D, Rubenstein L, Hirsch SH, et al. Value of functional status as a predictor of mortality: results of a prospective study. Am J Med 1992;93(6):663–9.

53. Landi F, Zuccalà G, Gambassi G, et al. Body mass index and mortality among older people living in the community. J Am Geriatr Soc 1999;47:1072.

54. Buccheri G, Ferrigno D, Tamburini M. Karnofsky and ECOG performance status scoring in lung cancer: a prospective, longitudinal study of 536 patients from a single institution. Eur J Cancer 1996;32A(7):1135–41.

55. Harpole DH Jr, Herndon JF 2nd, Young WG Jr, et al. Stage I nonsmall cell lung cancer: a multivariate analysis of treatment methods and patterns of recurrence. Cancer 1995;76:787–96.

56. Stamatis G, Djuric D, Eberhardt W, et al. Postoperative morbidity and mortality after induction chemoradiotherapy for locally advancer lung cancer: an analysis of 350 operated patients. Eur J Cardiothorac Surg 2002;22:292–7.

57. Ferguson MK, Vigneswaran WT. Diffusing capacity predicts morbidity after lung resection in patients without obstructive lung disease. Ann Thorac Surg 2008;85(4):1158–64.

58. Mery CM, Jaklitch MT. Lung resection in the elderly, correspondence. Chest 2006;129:496–7.

59. Albano WA. Should elderly patients undergo surgery for cancer. Geriatrics 1977;32:105–8.

60. Breyer RH, Zippe C, Pharr WF, et al. Thoracotomy in patients over age seventy years: ten-year experience. J Thorac Cardiovasc Surg 1981;81:187–93.

61. Zapatero J, Madrigal L, Lago J, et al. Thoracic Surgery in the elderly: review of 100 cases. Acta Chir Jung 1990;31:227–34.

62. Allen MS, Darling GE, Pechet TT, et al. ACOSOG Z0030 study group. Morbidity and mortality of major pulmonary resections in patients with early-stage lung cancer: initial results of the randomized, prospective ACOSOG Z0030 trial. Ann Thorac Surg 2006;81(3):1013–9.

Extended Chest Wall Resection and Reconstruction in the Setting of Lung Cancer

Daine T. Bennett, MD[a], Michael J. Weyant, MD[b],*

KEYWORDS

- Lung cancer • Chest wall resection • Reconstruction • Thorax

KEY POINTS

- En bloc, complete resection is mandatory.
- Defects less than 5 cm can be managed without large reconstruction.
- Larger anterior chest and sternal defects frequently need rigid prosthesis.
- With the wide range of reconstruction techniques available, materials should be selected to provide the best functional and cosmetic outcome.
- Involvement of multidisciplinary team, including plastic surgery and spine surgery when appropriate, is important.

INTRODUCTION

Chest wall resection and reconstruction remains a significant clinical dilemma in the setting of lung cancer. Although these lesions represent less than 10% of operable lung cancer in most series, the clinical challenges surrounding treatment of these lesions is significantly increased.[1] The addition of a chest wall resection to the surgical treatment of lung cancer magnifies the need for thorough staging and operative planning. The main determinants of survival after resection of these lesions are nodal involvement and completeness of resection.[1,2] The main factors attributed to the chance of postoperative morbidity include the size of the chest wall resection, extent of concomitant pulmonary resection, age, and underlying pulmonary function.[1–3]

Preoperative Diagnosis and Staging

Obtaining a tissue diagnosis of lesions that involve both the lung and chest wall simultaneously is important. Understanding the type of primary lung cancer and ruling out primary chest wall tumors that invade the lung help form the initial treatment plan. Imaging modalities such as computed tomography (CT) and 18-Fluoro-deoxyglucose positron emission tomography (FDG-PET) scanning assist in formulating a clinical stage of disease and are useful tools in the early stages of clinical decision making. Brain imaging is included in the preoperative evaluation of these patients given the higher likelihood of metastases in these locally advanced cancers.

Nodal staging is paramount in these patients. Given the locally advanced nature of these

Disclosure: The authors of this article have no relevant financial disclosures.
[a] Division of Cardiothoracic Surgery, Department of Surgery, University of Colorado Denver, School of Medicine, 12631 East 17th Avenue, MS 302, Aurora, CO 80045, USA; [b] Section of General Thoracic Surgery, Division of Cardiothoracic Surgery, University of Colorado Denver, School of Medicine, 12631 East 17th Avenue, MS C310, Aurora, CO 80045, USA
* Corresponding author.
E-mail address: michael.weyant@ucdenver.edu

Thorac Surg Clin 24 (2014) 383–390
http://dx.doi.org/10.1016/j.thorsurg.2014.07.002
1547-4127/14/$ – see front matter © 2014 Elsevier Inc. All rights reserved.

tumors, the chances of nodal involvement are also increased and significantly affect survival. The incidence of N2 nodal disease ranges from 15% to 21% in large series of T3 lung cancer.[1,2,4] The impact of N2 disease on overall survival is significant. The 5-year survival rate of node-negative patients is on average 40%. The overall survival rate of N2 disease ranges from 6% to 17%. This radical difference in survival rates suggests that great effort should be used in determining the nodal status of these patients. The technique of nodal evaluation has not been specifically studied in these patients; however, the routine use of surgical mediastinoscopy is our preferred technique.

Neoadjuvant Therapy

The only setting in which neoadjuvant therapy has been found to be beneficial is in regard to pancoast tumors. The important initial study by Rusch and colleagues[5] showing the benefit of neoadjuvant chemoradiotherapy in increasing the likelihood of obtaining negative margins in this subset of lung cancer patients established neoadjuvant chemoradiotherapy as the standard of care in patients with pancoast tumors. These findings should not be extrapolated to the treatment of other lung cancers that invade the chest wall, and en bloc resection should be considered the primary modality of treatment.

Most chest wall resections are performed because of malignancy, with the 3 main causes being primary chest wall tumors, non–small cell lung cancer (NSCLC), and breast cancer.[6–8] Perioperative mortality rates range from 2% to 7% with higher rates of morbidity. Inadequate reconstruction of extended chest wall resections has the potential to result in sternal instability or flail chest with subsequent respiratory compromise.

Preoperative Planning

Although mesh, methyl methacrylate, and soft tissue flaps have been used for the bulk of reconstruction, new therapeutic options developed in recent years continue to expand the available techniques for reconstruction. Titanium bars, bone autografts, and cryopreserved allografts are just a few of the novel techniques being applied to reconstruction of the chest wall.

When evaluating patients for potential chest wall resection, the surgeon must ensure that the underlying lesion has been adequately managed. Details of lesion-specific management are beyond the scope of this article. CT or magnetic resonance imaging is often adequate to determine the extent of tumor involvement. Standard preoperative work

should be performed to ensure the patient will tolerate the operation.

Careful assessment of imaging studies will find the extent and detailed location of the tumor. A multidisciplinary approach to management of the resection and reconstruction may be necessary. The spinal surgery department should be consulted when the planned area to be resected encroaches the vertebrae. For larger lesions that will potentially require a myocutaneous free flap, plastic surgery should also be involved in operative planning to assist with coverage. Postoperatively, the primary surgeon will undoubtedly work closely with the surgical intensivist for optimal postoperative management.

There are many approaches to managing chest wall lesions. This article addresses key principles of resection of malignant tumors of the chest well and the myriad of options for reconstructing these defects.

RESECTION AND SURGICAL TECHNIQUE
Surgical Technique

The location and size of the tumor will obviously dictate the surgical plan and approach. Preoperative imaging with CT is generally adequate to determine the extent of both the lung and chest wall resection required to remove the tumor. Occasionally, magnetic resonance imaging can help in providing information on encroachment into the vertebrae, which may require assistance and preoperative planning with spinal surgery. It is rare to observe a lung cancer that breaches the skin surface, and these findings should lead to a thorough evaluation of the initial diagnosis. Doddoli and colleagues report the need for muscle flap transfer in only 3 of 309 cases (1%).[2] If it is anticipated that a large skin surface will need to be resected, it is helpful to obtain consultation with a plastic surgeon.

Positioning and Incision

Most lung cancers with chest wall invasion can be approached via a thoracotomy in the lateral decubitus position. The exception to this is anterior pancoast tumors for which an anterior approach may be beneficial. The incision and interspace through which the thoracotomy is made should be carefully planned so as not to disrupt the tumor. This is done by carefully viewing the CT scan to determine the available interspaces. Alternatively, the use of video-assisted thoracoscopy has been described to aid in the decision-making part of this process. The video-assisted approach can also be used to inspect the pleura and look for signs of more advance disease.[9]

Chest Wall Resection

The order of whether the chest wall resection is performed initially or after the anatomic lung resection is not important as long as the entire specimen is removed en bloc. Resecting the chest wall before performing the anatomic lung resection is often the most practical approach, but on rare occasions, the anatomy presents itself such that the hilar dissection is more feasible to perform first.

The margins of resection are the most critical part of the en bloc resection. In 2 large series of NSCLC patients with tumors that invade the chest wall, R0 en bloc resection was found to improve 5-year survival with rates of 24% to 34% compared with incomplete resection being significantly lower, ranging from 13% to 14%.[4,10] There are no defined criteria for distance of the margin from the tumor akin to primary chest wall tumors. The technique we usually recommend is to make the inferior and superior margins the closest grossly uninvolved rib and the anterior and posterior margins transected through an area that is visually clear of tumor. Once the chest wall is free, multiple frozen sections are sent in circumferential fashion from the resection bed. The approach of performing the chest wall resection initially allows for efficiency of time, as the frozen sections may take time to analyze. The anatomic lung resection can then be performed during this period.

En Bloc Resection

En bloc resection provides better survival advantage. This may seem intuitive; however, in Doddoli and colleagues'[2] review of 309 cases of NSCLC invading the chest wall they found a 5-year survival advantage with en bloc resection over extrapleural mobilization in stage IIB NSCLC patients whose disease involved only the parietal pleura (60.3% vs 39.1%). This finding indicates that there is no precise method of determining the level of true chest wall invasion and that more aggressive, full-thickness chest wall resection is potentially favorable in most cases.

RECONSTRUCTION
General Considerations

Many aspects of the reconstruction of chest wall defects must be taken into consideration. Maintenance of anatomy, structural stability, and function must all be balanced to ensure the optimal outcome. Adequate material based on the size and location of the defect should be used to achieve a suitable final outcome.[6,7]

The reconstruction primarily protects the vital organs exposed by the rib resection. The return of structural stability in larger chest wall resections allows for preserved ventilatory mechanics. Achieving these goals will do the most to prevent pulmonary complications postoperatively. The need for reconstruction in cases of lung cancer is not ubiquitous, and in Doddoli's large series of chest wall resections for lung cancer, only 40% of patients had prosthetic reconstruction.[2] In general, anterior and lateral defects less than 5 cm and posterior defects less than 10 cm that are not at risk for scapular impingement are managed without rigid prostheses.[8] These smaller defects are adequately repaired with primary closure, mesh, local soft tissue, or a combination of these modalities. Larger defects will frequently require some type of rigid repair. Because of the potential paradoxic chest wall movement that ensues with larger chest wall defects, stabilization with a rigid prosthesis is recommended. Several options for rigid repairs will be discussed subsequently.

Specific anatomic and functional concerns vary depending on the location of the resected tumor. Larger sternal and anterior resections often necessitate rigid prostheses to stabilize the chest wall, although the need for this is rare in lung cancer patients, as primary lung tumors infrequently involve the sternum. Posterior resections of the uppermost ribs generally only require tissue or mesh coverage, because the large surface area of the scapula provides generous coverage over this area.[6]

Mesh Repair

When managing defects that do not result in significant chest wall instability, mesh alone allows for an acceptable repair. When dealing with a posterior defect that may result in scapular impingement, it is our practice to cover the defect with mesh. This is especially true with defects involving the fourth rib, because this is where the tip of the scapula usually rests (**Fig. 1**). The ideal mesh for repairing chest wall defects is tightly stretched across the defect to occlude the defect. Polytetrafluoroethylene (PTFE) mesh of 2-mm thickness or polypropylene mesh may be used in these instances. The mesh is stretched tight and secured with nonabsorbable suture around the ribs surrounding the defects.[8] It is important to note that most chest wall defects produced after resection of lung cancer can be managed using either PTFE or polypropylene mesh alone. The need occasionally arises in which large defects are created, and additional materials need to be used to reproduce the rigid chest wall. The standard approaches and newer novel materials that

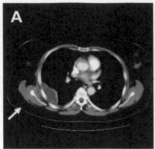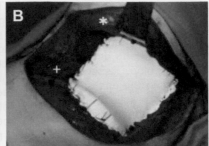

Fig. 1. (*A*) In situ tumor (*arrow*) invading the posterior chest wall. After resection, PTFE mesh is used to cover the defect (*B*) as the scapula (*asterisk*) is at risk of impinging behind the fourth rib (*plus*).

are available for reconstruction of the bony chest wall are described in later discussion.

Methyl Methacrylate

In a retrospective study of 262 patients undergoing chest wall reconstruction, Weyant and colleagues[3] found a decrease in postoperative pulmonary complications from the use of rigid prosthesis for larger defects. Methyl methacrylate is mixed into a resin and sized to fit the defect with a piece of polypropylene mesh incorporated into each side of the methyl methacrylate. Once the resin dries, the methyl methacrylate mesh sandwich is secured to the costal margins. The appropriate-size mold can be prepared on the back table in the operating room and then incorporated into the wound. An alternative method to this technique is pouring the resin in situ directly into the defect. This is done by securing a piece of mesh near the lung, pouring the resin onto the mesh, filling the defect and then incorporating another layer of mesh into the methyl methacrylate before it hardens. Lardinois and colleagues[11] found this technique to reduce the probability of dislodgement of the prosthesis.

Riblike Method

Girotti and colleagues[12] developed a novel technique to address the challenge of providing stability and coverage for sternal resections. Their riblike method uses an aluminum cast of the chest wall. The cast is covered by mesh, and then acrylic and methyl methacrylate resins are poured into the mold to fit the size of the defect. Once the reaction is hardened, the excess mesh is removed, and the mold is fixed to the costal stumps. In their series of 22 patients undergoing this technique, they noted only one respiratory complication, and no prostheses required removal. **Fig. 2** depicts this technique.

Titanium Ribs

Berthet and colleagues[13] recently described a technique for large chest wall defects. For their reconstructive technique, a 2-mm layer of PTFE is secured to the remaining ribs close to the lung parenchyma and stretched tight across the defect. Titanium implants (STRATOS, MedXpert GmbH; Heithersheim, Germany) are then inserted to bridge across the defect for structural integrity. This system involves a titanium anchor attached to each edge of the resected rib then bridged by a connecting titanium rod. A myocutaneous flap is mobilized to cover the synthetic implant. In their series of 19 patients, only 2 had infectious complications. Evaluation of pulmonary function tests before operation and 6 months after showed no significant reduction in forced expiratory volume in 1 second in the 14 patients evaluated. They did not observe any chest wall deformities. **Fig. 3** shows 3-dimensional reconstructed imaging of this system in place.

Biologics

Biologic implants encompass many alternative methods for reconstructing chest wall defects. Theses implants are especially useful for cases with high concerns for infection. Miller and colleagues[14] describe the use of bovine pericardial patches (Veritas, Synovis Life Technologies; St Paul, MN) with or without polylactic acid bars (Bio-Bridge, Acute Innovations; Hillsboro, OR). The bars are added when further structural stability is mandated (**Fig. 4**). In series of 25 patients, 10 of the patients had preoperatively infected resection sites, and none of these patients required excision of the implants postoperatively. The authors advocate the use of such biologic grafts for all infected sites as well as lateral chest wall defects and small sternal defects.

Another biologic option, which has recently been used to reconstruct large sternal defects, is

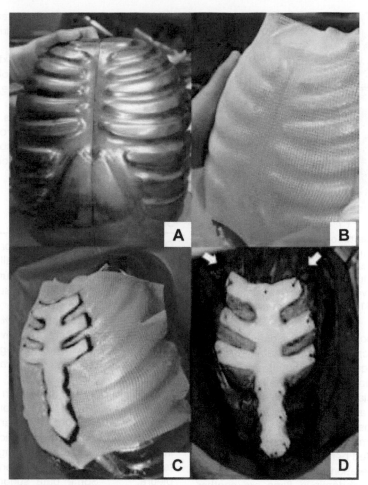

Fig. 2. The riblike prosthesis is modeled using (*A*) an aluminum cast that is (*B*) covered by a nonabsorbable mesh. (*C*) Cast tracks are filled over the mesh with radiopaque acrylic resin and methyl methacrylate resin. (*D*) Once the exothermic reaction is completed and redundant mesh is cut away, the prosthesis is washed and then fixed to the costal stumps. Clavicular stumps can also be fixed to the graft when required (*arrows*). (*From* Girotti P, Leo F, Bravi F, et al. The "rib-like" technique for surgical treatment of sternal tumors: lessons learned from 101 consecutive cases. Ann Thorac Surg 2011;92(4):1209. [discussion: 1215–6]; with permission.)

cryopreserved allografts.[15,16] These grafts are recovered from cadaveric donors, cleansed with antibiotic solution and stored at −80°C. When ready for implantation, the grafts thaw on ice and are tailored to fit the size of the defect. The grafts are secured with titanium plates and screws. Autologous costal and scapular grafts to reconstruct the chest wall have also been reported.[17,18] Although limited data are available on the outcomes for these techniques, it is an encouraging option for reconstruction of large defects.

Titanium Mesh

The use of titanium mesh was described in a case report by Suganuma and colleagues[19] to repair a chest wall defect involving the lateral third through sixth ribs. This technique uses a titanium micromesh that is sized to fill the defect plus at least one rib space on either side. The titanium micromesh is sandwiched between a layer of polyethylene mesh on either side. The mesh sandwich is secured to the surrounding ribs with titanium wires (**Fig. 5**). The titanium mesh is a porous titanium plate that is moderately malleable but also provides sufficient rigidity to prevent flail chest postoperatively.[19] This work, presented by Suganuma and colleagues[19] represents a novel technique applied to a single case with a good outcome but may be considered a feasible option for repairing an intermediate-sized chest wall defect.

Soft Tissue Coverage

Most chest wall defects after resection of an invading lung cancer can be covered primarily or

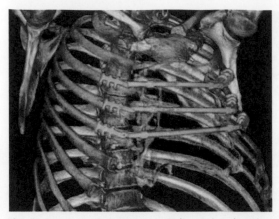

Fig. 3. Postoperative CT scan: 3-dimensional reconstruction after implantation of Strasbourg thoracic osteosynthesis system (STRATOS)/Dualmesh (3 bars). (*From* Berthet JP, Canaud L, D'Annoville T, et al. Titanium plates and Dualmesh: a modern combination for reconstructing very large chest wall defects. Ann Thorac Surg 2011;91(6):1711; with permission.)

with local advancement flaps alone. However, pedicle or free microvascular myocutaneous flaps are sometimes required for adequate coverage.

The myriad options for soft tissue flaps are well reviewed by Tukiainen[7] and Arnold and Pairolero.[20] For sternal and anterior chest wounds, pectoralis major flaps offer ideal coverage. When bilateral flaps are mobilized to adjoin in the midline, they offer the added benefit of not being compromised if future operations are required in the sternal area. Rectus abdominus flaps are another option to cover sternal and anterior wounds. The latissimus dorsi flap offers a broad range of coverage from the superior sternum to all areas of the chest wall and can be mobilized as a myocutaneous flap. External oblique mobilization

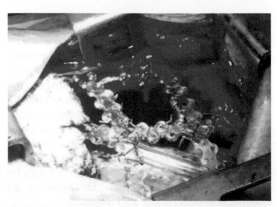

Fig. 4. Three BioBridge bars have been placed to reconstruct the posterior chest wall. (*From* Miller DL, Force SD, Pickens A, et al. Chest wall reconstruction using biomaterials. Ann Thorac Surg 2013;95(3):1051; with permission.)

adequately covers lower anteriolateral defects and is especially useful for repairing diaphragmatic wounds.

When resection results in extremely large defects or pedicled flaps are not a viable option because of damage or prior use, free myocutaneous flaps can be implemented. The tensor fascia lata with accompanying rectus femoris provides coverage for large defects. Prolonged operating time and risk of anastomotic complications must be taken into account when considering a free flap repair.

CLINICAL OUTCOMES
Survival (Lung Cancer)

Obtaining a complete resection in patients with NSCLC invading the chest wall improves 5-year survival. Matsuoka and colleagues[4] found a significant improvement in 5-year survival in patients with negative tissue margins (34%) compared with incomplete resection (14%), whereas depth of invasion did not affect survival. Similar results were found in a review by Magdeleinat and colleagues of 201 cases of lung cancer invading the chest wall.[10] Not surprisingly, many institutions have found poorer survival with increasing lymph node involvement.[1,4,21,22] The prognostic implications of the depth of invasion are divergent in the literature with some studies finding no difference in survival[2,4,21] and others finding a survival advantage when invasion is limited to the parietal pleura.[1,10,23] Some data suggest that adjuvant chemotherapy or radiotherapy improves 5-year survival; however, this appears to be dependent on the etiology of the tumor.[1,2,22]

Functional

Although few studies have evaluated postoperative functional data, Lardinois and colleagues[11] evaluated the 26 patients in their series who had defects involving 3 to 8 ribs with 39% of patients undergoing sternal resection. Using a mesh methyl methacrylate sandwich technique, they found no significant difference in preoperative and 6-month postoperative forced expiratory volume in 1 second. They also found concordant chest wall movement in 92% of patients by cine magnetic resonance imaging.

Complications and Concerns

Complication rates range from 24% to 46% based on larger retrospective reviews.[3,8,24,25] These studies span treatment periods of 1 to 2 decades, and undoubtedly care has improved over time. Although surgical technique has improved over

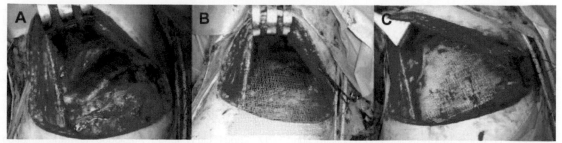

Fig. 5. Reconstruction of the left chest wall defect. (*A*) The left chest wall tumor was resected with the third to sixth ribs. (*B*) Titanium micromesh and Marlex mesh were appropriately cut larger than the skeletal defect. (*C*) Titanium micromesh covered with Marlex mesh was sutured to the second to eight ribs with titanium wires to improve rigidity. (*From* Suganuma N, Wada N, Arai H, et al. Chest wall resection and reconstruction using titanium micromesh covered with Marlex mesh for metastatic follicular thyroid carcinoma: a case report. J Med Case Rep 2009;3:7259; with permission.)

the years, complication rates remain high. Furthermore, perioperative mortality rates range from 2% to 7% in these studies. Wound (7%–19%) and pulmonary (7%–24%) complications are the most prevalent. Other complications include supraventricular arrhythmias, necrosis of soft tissue flap coverage, and removal of prosthesis.

With regard to pulmonary complications, a serious concern is postoperative flail chest and respiratory compromise caused by paradoxic movement of the chest wall from the inadequate repair of a large defect. Repairing anterior defects greater than 5 cm with a structural repair including mesh and rigid prosthesis reduces the risk of this complication. Mesh repairs must be secured with the mesh taught across the chest wall defect to prevent paradoxic movement.

Involving mesh or rigid prosthesis into the reconstruction introduces a foreign body into the patient with higher chances for postoperative infection. For wounds that are contaminated at the time of operation, consideration should be given to using a biologic alternative. In a subset of 10 patients with contaminated wounds at resection, Miller and colleagues[14] found no postoperative wound complications using bovine pericardial patches and polylactic acid bars for repair. Although this was a small group of patients, it is an alternative technique to consider when managing a contaminated space.

Seroma formation has been seen in up to 7% of patients. Placing drains at the time of operation and leaving them until daily output is less than 25 mL/d may reduce the risk of seroma formation. Small seromas frequently resolve spontaneously. Large or symptomatic seromas can be treated by repeated aseptic aspirations. Rarely, reoperation with surgical obliteration of space may be required.[8]

Lans and colleagues[25] evaluated causes of wound healing complications in 220 undergoing chest wall resection and reconstruction. They found that ulceration of the tumor and use of omental flap for tissue coverage resulted in wound healing complications.

SUMMARY

Reconstruction of large chest wall defects after resection remains a significant undertaking. Obtaining a negative margin is of paramount importance for long-term survival. While reconstructing the chest wall, recreating a stable chest wall with adequate functional capacity and reasonable cosmesis are always the end goals. Morbidity from these procedures is significant, and mortality continues to hover around 5%. With continued advancement in reconstructive techniques and improved perioperative management, these procedures will continue to result in improved outcomes for patients.

REFERENCES

1. Facciolo F, Cardillo G, Lopergolo M, et al. Chest wall invasion in non-small cell lung carcinoma: a rationale for en bloc resection. J Thorac Cardiovasc Surg 2001;121(4):649–56. http://dx.doi.org/10.1067/mtc. 2001.112826.

2. Doddoli C, D'Journo B, Le Pimpec-Barthes F, et al. Lung cancer invading the chest wall: a plea for en-bloc resection but the need for new treatment strategies. Ann Thorac Surg 2005;80(6):2032–40. http:// dx.doi.org/10.1016/j.athoracsur.2005.03.088.

3. Weyant MJ, Bains MS, Venkatraman E, et al. Results of chest wall resection and reconstruction with and without rigid prosthesis. Ann Thorac Surg 2006; 81(1):279–85. http://dx.doi.org/10.1016/j.athoracsur. 2005.07.001.

4. Matsuoka H, Nishio W, Okada M, et al. Resection of chest wall invasion in patients with non-small cell lung

cancer. Eur J Cardiothorac Surg 2004;26(6):1200–4. http://dx.doi.org/10.1016/j.ejcts.2004.07.038.

5. Rusch VW, Giroux DJ, Kraut MJ, et al. Induction chemoradiation and surgical resection for superior sulcus non-small-cell lung carcinomas: long-term results of Southwest Oncology Group Trial 9416 (Intergroup Trial 0160). J Clin Oncol 2007; 25(3):313–8. http://dx.doi.org/10.1200/JCO.2006. 08.2826.

6. Rocco G. Chest wall resection and reconstruction according to the principles of biomimesis. Semin Thorac Cardiovasc Surg 2011;23(4):307–13. http:// dx.doi.org/10.1053/j.semtcvs.2012.01.011.

7. Tukiainen E. Chest wall reconstruction after oncological resections. Scand J Surg 2013;102(1):9–13. Available at: http://www.ncbi.nlm.nih.gov/pubmed/ 23628630.

8. Deschamps C, Tirnaksiz BM, Darbandi R, et al. Early and long-term results of prosthetic chest wall reconstruction. J Thorac Cardiovasc Surg 1999;117(3): 588–91 [discussion: 591–2]. Available at: http:// www.ncbi.nlm.nih.gov/pubmed/10047664.

9. Demmy TL, Yendamuri S, Hennon MW, et al. Thoracoscopic maneuvers for chest wall resection and reconstruction. J Thorac Cardiovasc Surg 2012; 144(3):S52–7. http://dx.doi.org/10.1016/j.jtcvs.2012. 06.005.

10. Magdeleinat P, Alifano M, Benbrahem C, et al. Surgical treatment of lung cancer invading the chest wall: results and prognostic factors. Ann Thorac Surg 2001;71(4):1094–9. Available at: http://www.ncbi. nlm.nih.gov/pubmed/11308142.

11. Lardinois D, Müller M, Furrer M, et al. Functional assessment of chest wall integrity after methylmethacrylate reconstruction. Ann Thorac Surg 2000; 69(3):919–23. Available at: http://www.ncbi.nlm.nih. gov/pubmed/10750784.

12. Girotti P, Leo F, Bravi F, et al. The "rib-like" technique for surgical treatment of sternal tumors: lessons learned from 101 consecutive cases. Ann Thorac Surg 2011;92(4):1208–15. http://dx.doi.org/10.1016/ j.athoracsur.2011.05.016 [discussion: 1215–6].

13. Berthet JP, Canaud L, D'Annoville T, et al. Titanium plates and Dualmesh: a modern combination for reconstructing very large chest wall defects. Ann Thorac Surg 2011;91(6):1709–16. http://dx.doi.org/ 10.1016/j.athoracsur.2011.02.014.

14. Miller DL, Force SD, Pickens A, et al. Chest wall reconstruction using biomaterials. Ann Thorac Surg 2013; 95(3):1050–6. http://dx.doi.org/10.1016/j.athoracsur. 2012.11.024.

15. Marulli G, Hamad AM, Cogliati E, et al. Allograft sternochondral replacement after resection of large sternal chondrosarcoma. J Thorac Cardiovasc Surg 2010; 139(4):e69–70. http://dx.doi.org/10.1016/j.jtcvs.2009. 01.007.

16. Rocco G, Fazioli F. Cryopreserved biomaterials for chest wall reconstruction. Multimed Man Cardiothorac Surg 2009;2009(209):6–8. http://dx.doi.org/ 10.1510/mmcts.2008.003277.

17. Zhou F, Liu W, Tang Y. Autologous rib transplantation and terylene patch for repair of chest wall defect in a girl with Poland syndrome: a case report. J Pediatr Surg 2008;43(10):1902–5. http://dx.doi.org/10.1016/ j.jpedsurg.2008.06.005.

18. Prantl L, Gehmert S, Nerlich M, et al. Successful reconstruction of sternum with a scapular autograft segment: 5-year follow-up. Ann Thorac Surg 2011; 92(5):1889–91. http://dx.doi.org/10.1016/j.athoracsur. 2011.04.070.

19. Suganuma N, Wada N, Arai H, et al. Chest wall resection and reconstruction using titanium micromesh covered with Marlex mesh for metastatic follicular thyroid carcinoma: a case report. J Med Case Rep 2009;3:7259. http://dx.doi.org/10.4076/ 1752-1947-3-7259.

20. Arnold PG, Pairolero PC. Chest-wall reconstruction: an account of 500 consecutive patients. Plast Reconstr Surg 1996;98:804–10.

21. Lin YT, Hsu PK, Hsu HS, et al. En bloc resection for lung cancer with chest wall invasion. J Chin Med Assoc 2006;69(4):157–61. http://dx.doi.org/10.1016/ S1726-4901(09)70197-2.

22. Lee CY, Byun CS, Lee JG, et al. The prognostic factors of resected non-small cell lung cancer with chest wall invasion. World J Surg Oncol 2012; 10(1):9. http://dx.doi.org/10.1186/1477-7819-10-9.

23. Chapelier A, Fadel E, Macchiarini P, et al. Factors affecting long-term survival after en-bloc resection of lung cancer invading the chest wall. Eur J Cardiothorac Surg 2000;18(5):513–8. Available at: http:// www.ncbi.nlm.nih.gov/pubmed/11053809.

24. Mansour KA, Thourani VH, Losken A, et al. Chest wall resections and reconstruction: a 25-year experience. Ann Thorac Surg 2002;73(6):1720–5 [discussion: 1725–6]. Available at: http://www.ncbi.nlm.nih. gov/pubmed/12078759.

25. Lans TE, van der Pol C, Wouters MW, et al. Complications in wound healing after chest wall resection in cancer patients; a multivariate analysis of 220 patients. J Thorac Oncol 2009;4(5):639–43. http://dx. doi.org/10.1097/JTO.0b013e31819d18c9.

The Management of Non–Small Cell Lung Cancer With Oligometastases

Robert J. Downey, MD

KEYWORDS

• Lung cancer • Oligometastases • Surgery • Chemotherapy • Survival

KEY POINTS

• Effective treatment in patients with oligometastatic spread requires:
  ○ The ability to eradicate the primary site.
  ○ The ability to image all sites of metastatic disease.
  ○ The ability to ablate all evident metastatic sites.
  ○ Effective systemic therapy to eradicate undetectable micrometastatic disease.

INTRODUCTION

The standard of care for patients with non–small cell lung cancer (NSCLC) with hematogenous metastases is either chemotherapy or supportive care, with surgery or other ablative therapy reserved for palliation of symptoms. A small number of patients with NSCLC have a limited number of extrathoracic metastases (oligometastases); these patients are currently offered resection of both the metastases and the primary site, plus or minus systemic treatment, with the goal of extending survival and possibly curing patients. Only limited data are available addressing the efficacy and safety of such an approach, but the results published to date support continued investigation. In this article, the author first summarizes the theoretic and clinical bases for resecting oligometastatic cancer of the lung and other histologic types; second, the author reviews the published data, addressing the specific question of management of lung cancer that is metastatic to the lung, the brain, and the adrenal gland; and third, the author suggests an outline of possible clinical trials to further investigate the management of oligometastatic NSCLC.

BACKGROUND

The pioneering surgeon William Stewart Halsted[1] held that malignant disease spreads in an orderly fashion from the primary site, through the regional lymphatics, to systemic sites, suggesting that, in the absence of evidence of distant metastases, the surgeon should offer extensive local exenteration. Since then, others have held the opposing view that metastatic spread, even if only to the lymphatics, connotes a high probability of diffuse systemic metastases; therefore, surgical removal of the metastases will be of very limited benefit, as progression at undetected distant sites will determine survival.

If these models are seen as mutually exclusive, it is unlikely that either encompasses the varieties of malignancy. The emerging model of cancer is built on the belief that the human body is a remarkable example of coordinated and well-regulated multicellularity, such that diverse cell types respond to external signals to differentiate, as needed, but also to undergo apoptosis if directed by internal or external signals. The need for each cell to participate in the functioning of the overall multicellular organism is so great that the pathways

Disclosure: The author has no relevant conflicts of interest.
Thoracic Service, Department of Surgery, Memorial Hospital, Memorial Sloan Kettering Cancer Center, 1275 York Avenue, New York, NY 10021, USA
E-mail address: downeyr@mskcc.org

Thorac Surg Clin 24 (2014) 391–397
http://dx.doi.org/10.1016/j.thorsurg.2014.07.003
1547-4127/14/$ – see front matter © 2014 Elsevier Inc. All rights reserved.

thoracic.theclinics.com

regulating proliferation and apoptosis are multiple and overlapping. The problem, leading to cancer, is that all cells accumulate random mutations during cell division; unfortunately, there will amass a subpopulation of cells with accumulations of random mutations, resulting in inactivation of the pathways that regulate proliferation and apoptosis and effecting a rogue cell that benefits from the nutrition, oxygen, and waste-disposal mechanisms (among other features) of the host but that is free from external regulation and so proliferates and disseminates in an uncontrolled fashion. Associated with the loss of these regulatory pathways is the emergence of the multiple attributes of malignancy, primarily the avoidance of immune surveillance; local invasiveness; the ability to break into and survive within the blood and/or lymph systems; and the ability to assume residence, survive, and grow within a new host organ.

It is clear that cancers—even histologically similar ones originating from the same organ—fall along a spectrum of malignancy, ranging from, at one end, indolent disease likely to remain localized to, at the other end, highly aggressive disease featuring local growth that is rapid, invasive, and associated with the appearance of multiple sites of metastasis within multiple distant organs. How cancers are distributed along this spectrum of aggressive behavior (how many and specifically which regulatory pathways have been disabled) remains an open question. More specifically, although it is beyond the scope of this review, it is likely that, rather than being evenly distributed along a spectrum of malignant disease, cancers cluster at certain points on this spectrum, allowing for the distinction of cancers into 2 main groups: (1) cancers with indolent behavior, for which, even if oligometastatic disease is present, treatment should comprise ablative therapies[2] and (2) cancers with an essentially complete loss of regulatory control and, therefore, such aggressive potential that the development of diffuse systemic metastasis is essentially inevitable and for which only systemic therapies should be used.

Evidence that a curable oligometastatic disease state exists is largely only available for malignancies other than lung cancer. In general, there are 2 ways that such a curable state could be reached: a malignancy may, at the time of diagnosis, be found to have spread to only a limited number of sites and, alternatively, a malignancy with extensive systemic spread may be reduced to a limited number of sites by effective systemic therapy. Nonlung examples of the former include sarcoma[3,4] and colorectal cancer,[5] both of which spread to the lung as isolated sites of metastatic disease; in such cases, lung resection seems to offer patients an improved likelihood of prolonged survival. An example of the second form is germ cell tumors, for which resection of residual disease remaining after chemotherapy offers improved survival, compared with nonsurgical therapy alone.[6]

In patients with oligometastatic spread, effective treatment requires multiple capabilities: first, the ability to eradicate the primary site; second, the ability to image all sites of metastatic disease; third, the ability to ablate all evident metastatic sites; and fourth, effective systemic therapy to eradicate undetectable micrometastatic disease. Therefore, as the ability to achieve all 4 of these goals will differ depending on the particular disease under consideration, the likelihood that oligometastatic lung cancer can be considered curable by the successes with other histologic types should be considered weak.

EXTENT OF THE PROBLEM: PERCENTAGE OF PATIENTS WITH NON–SMALL CELL LUNG CANCER WITH OLIGOMETASTATIC DISEASE

For the purposes of this article, the author considers oligometastatic disease to consist of disease that includes a solitary hematogenous metastasis in a single extrathoracic organ. The number of patients with lung cancer with such an oligometastatic state is not clear. At the time of autopsy (and, presumably, most often after unsuccessful treatment of disease), distant metastases are found in up to 93% of patients, with the major sites of metastases being liver, bone, skin, adrenal glands, brain, and abdominal lymph nodes.[7] Estimates of the frequency of M_1 disease at the time of the initial diagnosis are lower. In a prospective study of 146 patients with radiographically resectable intrathoracic disease without symptoms of hematogenous metastatic disease, Salvatierra and colleagues[8] found that brain computed tomography (CT) scan, abdominal ultrasound, and bone scan detected extrathoracic metastases in 44 patients (30%); 27 of these cases were apparently solitary, and 17 were multiple. In another study, limited to patients imaged with thoracic CT scans (which suggests that these patients had resectable intrathoracic disease with normal mediastinal lymph nodes),[9] extrathoracic sites of disease were found in 25% of patients; the investigators did not provide information on how many of these M_1 sites were solitary. Finally, in a detailed analysis of newly diagnosed patients staged by means of imaging studies, all of whom underwent CT scans of the chest and upper abdomen, with other imaging studies, such as abdominal CT scans, bone scans, and/or brain CT scans or magnetic resonance imaging (MRI) obtained either at the discretion of the caring physicians or if indicated by symptoms, Quint and colleagues[10] found M_1 disease in 21% of patients, with approximately two-thirds of cases isolated to a single body part (brain, 29%; bone, 25%; liver, 14%; adrenal glands, 6%; lung, 12%; body wall, 6%; other sites, 8%). This study was limited in that the routine addition of bone and brain imaging or a positron emission tomography (PET) scan[11] would likely have resulted in the detection of more sites of metastatic disease.

Limited metastatic disease may also become evident in the period following the treatment of intrathoracic disease. Figlin and colleagues[12] found that, of 1532 patients who had undergone apparently complete resection of NSCLC, 550 (36%) had a solitary site of the first recurrence (brain, 18%; ipsilateral lung, 18%; contralateral lung, 9%; bone, 14%; mediastinum, 6%; skin, 4% lymph nodes and 1% skin).

THE PRESENT

The best evidence to date that a curable oligometastatic disease state exists for lung cancer largely derives from the survival data on retrospective patients who have undergone surgical resection of a solitary M_1 site and all intrathoracic disease. Recently, a systematic review of the available literature was performed.[13] The investigators identified 49 studies comprising 2176 patients who met their eligibility criteria, which can be summarized as NSCLC with 1 to 5 metastases treated with either surgical metastasectomy or radiation therapy. The overall survival for patients in whom the primary site was controlled was 19 months. Highly significant prognostic factors included the achievement of definitive treatment of the primary site of disease, nodal status, and a disease-free interval of 6 to 12 months. The investigators noted that the patients included in the reviewed series were likely highly selected in that they had controllable primary sites of disease, had 1 to 3 metastases (most often in the brain), were of relatively young age, and had good performance status.

Most published case series have focused on cerebral and adrenal metastases. Although reports detailing the management of other M_1 sites have been published (including small bowel,[14–16] spleen,[17,18] lymph nodes, skeletal muscle, and bone[19]), the available data are too scant to allow strong conclusions to be made. A meta-analysis was recently performed on the subgroup of patients with a limited number of metastases to organs other than the adrenal glands and the brain.[20] Sixty-two cases were identified. The 5-year survival was 50%, with the presence of mediastinal

nodal disease being an indicator of very poor prognosis. It is important to note that metastases to different organs should not necessarily be considered equivalent; in other words, even if it were shown that adrenal metastases could be treated with curative intent, this should not be considered strong evidence that brain metastases are also curable. The differences between sites include the feasibility of wide surgical resection (obviously limited with cerebral disease), the penetration of chemotherapy to the site to eradicate residual micrometastatic disease, and the likelihood that the clones of cells giving rise to metastases in different organs are fundamentally different. For example, adrenal metastases diagnosed as a solitary site of disease have been held to represent lymphatic dissemination rather than hematogenous spread[21]; furthermore, the clones of lung cancer cells that form lymphatic metastases likely represent less virulent disease than clones that form hematogenous metastases.[22]

LUNG METASTASES

The contralateral lung is an uncommon site of metastatic disease: In 2 autopsy studies on patients who died of lung cancer, contralateral disease was found in 20% and 22% of patients, respectively.[23,24] If 2 lesions are of similar histologic types, it can be difficult or even impossible to determine whether they are synchronous primaries or whether one is the primary and the other a metastasis. Martini and Melamed[25] suggested that, when 2 foci of NSCLC disease are noted in the lungs, they should be treated as synchronous primaries if the lesions are (1) physically distinct and separate; (2) in different segments, lobes, or lungs; (3) associated with carcinoma in situ; (4) without metastases to the lymphatics in common; and (5) without extrapulmonary metastases. Using these guidelines,[25] estimates of the incidence of synchronous primary lung cancer range from 0.26%[26] to 1.33%.[27] Given these data, until a method becomes available that can clearly differentiate synchronous primary from oligometastatic disease, it is reasonable to give patients the benefit of the doubt and treat the 2 lesions as 2 primaries. In such cases, the outcome achieved by surgery can be estimated to be equivalent to that for the lesion with the worst prognosis, minus 10%.[28–30] The causes that contribute to this poorer prognosis include the propensity for patients to develop further cancers, limited resections being performed more frequently than would be performed for a single site of disease, and/or the probability that some of these lesions are in fact metastases and not second primaries.

CEREBRAL METASTASES

Brain metastases are clinically evident in 30% of patients with NSCLC and are found at autopsy in 50%.[12] The median survival for patients with an untreated cerebral metastasis is 1 month.[31] Steroid therapy increases the median survival to 2 months, and whole-brain irradiation increases it to 3 to 8 months.

At the time of the initial diagnosis of lung cancer, intracranial metastases are diagnosed in 10% or less of cases. However, cerebral metastases are present in almost a third of patients with newly diagnosed NSCLC with solitary M_1 sites of disease.[10] After an apparently complete resection of a stage I to III lung cancer, 10% to 20% of patients will experience a first recurrence in the brain, with 94% of these recurrences being solitary.

As noted earlier, the prognosis of untreated brain metastases is dismal, with a median survival of 1 month. In 1926, Grant[32] reviewed 49 patients with brain metastases and stated that "surgery is of no ultimate benefit as far as prolongation of life is concerned"[32]; because of this view, the treatment of brain metastases was initially limited to steroids and irradiation. These methods proved to be of limited benefit, with median survivals of only 3 to 6 months.[33] Improved neurosurgical techniques have led to renewed and successful attempts at resection of brain metastases; in 1986, 2 retrospective series, by Mandell and colleagues[34] and Patchell and colleagues,[35] showed that resection of cerebral metastasis followed by whole-brain irradiation improved survival, compared with irradiation alone. These results were confirmed in 2 subsequent prospective trials.[36,37]

The first large series of patients subjected to combined resection of synchronous solitary cerebral metastasis and primary pulmonary neoplasm was published by Magilligan and colleagues[38,39] in 1976, with an update of 41 patients in 1986. Twenty-five of the patients also received cranial radiation, and 5 received chemotherapy. Survival was 55% at 1 year, 21% at 5 years, and 15% at 10 years. Since then, other groups have published similar results. In 1989, Read and colleagues[40] found survival rates after combined pulmonary and brain resection of 52% at 1 year and 21% at 5 years; in 1999, Saitoh and colleagues[41] reported 3- and 5-year survivals of 12% and 8% after combined resection. Finally, an analysis of the Memorial Sloan Kettering Cancer Center experience, which was published by Burt and colleagues[42] in 1992, with 65 patients with NSCLC, and updated by Wronski and colleagues[43] in 1995, with patients undergoing complete resection of intracranial disease of diverse histologic types, including 185 patients with primary lung cancer, found a median survival of 27 months if the intrathoracic disease was resectable and 11 months if it was not.

Recently published retrospective studies continue to suggest that, in patients with oligometastatic NSCLC involving the brain, there may be a survival advantage for ablative therapy to all sites of disease. Collaud and colleagues[44] performed a retrospective single-center review of 29 patients, of whom 19 had intracranial metastases. Patients with resected brain metastases had a 5-year survival of 37%. Griffioen and colleagues[45] performed a 2-center retrospective review of 50 patients with solitary extrathoracic metastases from NSCLC, of whom 36 had intracranial metastases. The overall survival for the subgroup of patients with brain metastases was 22 months.

Taken together, the findings of the available retrospective series suggest that, after complete resection of both the primary lung lesion and the cerebral metastasis, possibly in combination with other treatments, such as chemotherapy and whole-brain radiation therapy, a 1-year survival of 50% and a 5-year survival of 10% to 30% can be expected.

ADRENAL METASTASES

Adrenal metastases are found at autopsy in greater than 30% of patients.[46] At the time of the initial diagnosis of an otherwise operable lung cancer, the frequency of isolated adrenal metastases is estimated to range from 1.6% to 6.0%.[10,47]

Multiple retrospective series of patients who have undergone surgical management of a primary lung cancer with a solitary adrenal metastasis have been published; there are essentially no published prospective data, with the exception of the results from a Memorial Sloan Kettering Cancer Center trial, discussed later, which included only 3 patients with adrenal metastases. Eleven retrospective papers were analyzed in a collective review published by Beitler and colleagues[48] in 1998, which included a total of 60 patients, 32 of whom had sufficient data available for analysis. Adrenal metastases were synchronous in 59% of patients. The stage of locoregional disease was I in 22% of patients, II in 16%, III in 43%, and not specified in 18%. The median survival was 24 months, with approximately 30% of patients surviving 5 years. These data are obviously limited, as they are subject to the usual potential biases of retrospective reviews and the patients were treated for many different stages of locoregional disease, with and without the addition of chemotherapy or radiation therapy. Nevertheless, the Memorial Sloan Kettering Cancer Center retrospective experience[49] (included in the aforementioned review) found that the median survival of patients with adrenal metastases treated with chemotherapy alone was approximately 8.5 months, with all patients dead by 21 months; the survival of patients treated with chemotherapy and surgical resection of all known disease was 31 months (with 2 long-term survivors).

COMPLETED CLINICAL TRIALS

Following the improved results with the addition of surgical resection, the author and colleagues completed, at the Memorial Sloan Kettering Cancer Center, a phase II trial of induction therapy followed by resection of all sites of disease for patients with histologically proven lung cancer and a solitary M_1 site.[50] The largest subgroup of M_1 sites was intracranial. Of the 23 patients enrolled in the study, 14 had intracranial disease, which was resected when diagnosed in all patients, with adjuvant cranial radiation therapy used in 9 patients (64%). The stage of locoregional disease for the 14 patients was IIIA in 9 patients (64%) and IB in 5 patients (36%). Eleven of the 14 patients (79%) completed more than 2 cycles of induction therapy, and 29% had a response. Surgical resection of all intrathoracic disease was performed in 7 patients, with no operative deaths; the other patients either had progression in the chest ($n = 2$) or the brain ($n = 1$) or were without radiological evidence of a response to chemotherapy and, therefore, resection was not attempted ($n = 4$). The median survival of all 14 patients with cerebral metastases was 9 months, with 1 patient with locoregional stage IB disease who underwent pulmonary resection surviving for greater than 27 months.

Overall, the addition of surgical resection of the primary lung tumor and the M_1 sites for all patients enrolled resulted in survival rates similar to those for patients treated with chemotherapy or radiation therapy alone (5-year overall survival, 8%; disease-free survival, 4%). A review of the literature does not reveal any other published prospective series of patients undergoing combined modality therapy for a primary lung tumor and solitary M_1 disease. Phase II trials have been attempted for patients with oligometastatic NSCLC. The first trial (NCT0887315) randomized patients with 5 or fewer metastases after chemotherapy to receive either radiation therapy to all sites of disease or ongoing chemotherapy. The second trial (NCT00776100) randomized patients with 3 or fewer metastases after chemotherapy to receive either radiation therapy to all sites of disease or observation. Both trials closed because of poor patient accrual.

FUTURE DIRECTIONS

The limited information available suggests that there may be a small group of patients with primary lung cancer with a solitary extrathoracic site of metastatic disease who would benefit from therapy other than systemic chemotherapy alone. Whether this treatment would best consist of surgical resection of both sites of disease without chemotherapy or resection in combination with chemotherapy and/or radiation therapy cannot be determined from the available information. Given the recent unsuccessful attempts at prospective randomized trials, efforts should probably be directed toward single- or multi-institution efforts to accrue sufficient patients to complete a phase II trial.

A trial should require standardized staging and therapy as well as stratification for locoregional stage and the site of extrathoracic metastasis (perhaps a realistic approach would be cerebral vs all other sites combined). Separate algorithms for synchronous and metachronous disease could be considered.

Synchronous disease
1. Histologic confirmation of a primary NSCLC
2. Radiographic staging that suggests a solitary site of extrathoracic metastatic spread, by use of CT scans of the chest and upper abdomen, brain MRIs, and PET scans, with other imaging studies obtained as indicated by physical examination, history, or abnormalities on the aforementioned imaging studies
3. Histologic confirmation of the presence of an M_1 site that is consistent with the primary lung malignancy by means of needle aspiration or surgical excision
4. Bronchoscopy and mediastinal staging (by endobronchial ultrasound guided needle biopsy, mediastinoscopy, or mediastinotomy) for locoregional staging, with patients removed from consideration for surgical resection by use of the same criteria used in the absence of M_1 disease (for example, carinal involvement, N_3 disease, or multiple bulky nodal metastases)
5. Induction chemotherapy
6. Restaging by use of studies similar to those listed earlier, with patients with progression of disease being removed from study
7. Definitive ablation of metastatic sites, which may be either at presentation, if necessary (ie, symptomatic brain metastases or boney lesion with imminent fracture), or after induction chemotherapy and with or without radiation therapy, as deemed appropriate
8. Surgical resection of residual disease at the primary site

A similar algorithm for the management of patients with metachronous metastases could be as follows:

Metachronous disease
1. Histologic confirmation of a primary NSCLC within the previous 5 years
2. Radiographic staging that suggests a solitary site of extrathoracic metastatic spread, by use of CT scans of the chest and upper abdomen, brain MRIs, and PET scans, with other imaging studies obtained as indicated by physical examination, history, or findings on the aforementioned radiographic studies
3. Definitive ablation of the metastatic site by surgery, with or without radiation therapy, as deemed appropriate, with either neoadjuvant or adjuvant chemotherapy

Should the multimodality treatment in this trial fail to significantly improve survival over that achieved by chemotherapy alone, consideration should be given to a subsequent trial investigating the possibility that surgical resection of the locoregional disease and the solitary site of metastatic disease, without chemotherapy, might provide an opportunity for extended disease-free survival, similar to that achieved with chemotherapy alone.

SUMMARY

In the absence of persuasive findings from the trials outlined earlier, the available evidence supports treating patients with a solitary site of M_1 disease with induction chemotherapy followed by resection of all sites of disease as long as patients understand that this multimodality approach has not been proven to be superior to either surgery alone or chemotherapy alone.

REFERENCES

1. Halsted WS. The results of radical operations for the cure of carcinoma of the breast. Ann Surg 1907;46: 1–19.
2. Hellman S, Weichselbaum RR. Oligometastases. J Clin Oncol 1995;13(1):8–10.
3. Billingsley KG, Burt ME, Jara E, et al. Pulmonary metastases from soft tissue sarcoma: analysis of patterns of diseases and postmetastasis survival. Ann Surg 1999;229(5):602–10.
4. Billingsley KG, Lewis JJ, Leung DH, et al. Multifactorial analysis of the survival of patients with distant metastasis arising from primary extremity sarcoma. Cancer 1999;15(85):389–95.
5. Fong Y, Salo J. Surgical therapy of hepatic colorectal metastasis. Semin Oncol 1999;26:514–23.
6. Sheinfeld J, Bajorin D. Management of the postchemotherapy residual mass. Urol Clin North Am 1993;20:133–43.
7. Abrams HL, Spiro R, Goldstein N. Metastases in carcinoma. Analysis of 1000 autopsied cases. Cancer 1950;3:74–85.
8. Salvatierra A, Baamonde C, Llamas JM, et al. Extrathoracic staging of bronchogenic carcinoma. Chest 1990;97:1052–8.
9. Sider L, Horejs D. Frequency of extrathoracic metastases from bronchogenic carcinoma in patients with normal-sized hilar and mediastinal lymph nodes on CT. AJR Am J Roentgenol 1998;151:893–5.
10. Quint LE, Tummala S, Brisson LJ, et al. Distribution of distant metastases from newly diagnosed non-small cell lung cancer. Ann Thorac Surg 1996;62:246–50.
11. Erasmus JJ, Patz EF, McAdams HP, et al. Evaluation of adrenal masses in patients with bronchogenic carcinoma using 18F-fluorodeoxyglucose positron emission tomography. AJR Am J Roentgenol 1997;168:1357–60.
12. Figlin RA, Piantadosi S, Feld R, The Lung Cancer Study Group. Intracranial recurrence of carcinoma after complete surgical resection of stage I, II, and III non-small-cell lung cancer. N Engl J Med 1988; 318:1300–5.
13. Ashworth A, Rodrigues G, Boldt G, et al. Is there a oligometastatic state in non-small cell lung cancer? A systematic review of the literature. Lung Cancer 2013;82:197–203.
14. Hinoshita E, Nakahashi H, Wakasugi K, et al. Duodenal metastasis from large cell carcinoma of the lung: report of a case. Surg Today 1999;29(8): 799–802.
15. Berger A, Cellier C, Daniel C, et al. Small bowel metastases from primary carcinoma of the lung: clinical findings and outcome. Am J Gastroenterol 1999;94(7):1884–7.
16. Mosier DM, Bloch RS, Cunningham PL, et al. Small bowel metastases from primary lung carcinoma: a rarity waiting to be found? Am Surg 1992;58:677–82.
17. Macheers SK, Mansour KA. Management of isolated splenic metastases from carcinoma of the lung: a case report and review of the literature. Am Surg 1992;58:683–5.
18. Edelman AS, Rotterdam H. Solitary splenic metastasis of an adenocarcinoma of the lung. Am J Clin Pathol 1990;94:326–8.
19. Luketich JD, Martini N, Ginsberg RJ, et al. Successful treatment of solitary extracranial metastases from non-small cell lung cancer. Ann Thorac Surg 1995;60:1609–11.
20. Salah S, Tanvetyanon T, Abbasi S. Metastasectomy for extra-cranial non-small cell lung cancer solitary metastases: systematic review and analysis of reported cases. Lung Cancer 2012;75:9–14.

21. Karolyi P. Do adrenal metastases from lung cancer develop by lymphogenous or hematogenous route? J Surg Oncol 1990;43:154–6.

22. Nomori H, Nakajima T, Noguchi M, et al. Cytofluoro-metric analysis of metastases from lung adenocarcinoma with special reference to the difference between hematogenous and lymphatic metastases. Cancer 1991;67:2941–7.

23. Onuigbo WI. Contralateral pulmonary metastases in lung cancer. Thorax 1974;29:132–3.

24. Muir CS. Cancer of the lung, trachea and larynx in Singapore. Br J Cancer 1960;14:1–7.

25. Martini N, Melamed MR. Multiple primary lung cancers. J Thorac Cardiovasc Surg 1975;20:606–12.

26. Wu SC, Lin ZQ, Xu CW, et al. Multiple primary lung cancers. Chest 1987;92:892–6.

27. Ferguson MK, DeMeester TR, DesLauriers J, et al. Diagnosis and management of synchronous lung cancers. J Thorac Cardiovasc Surg 1985;89:378–85.

28. Rosengart TK, Martini N, Ghosn P, et al. Multiple primary lung carcinoma: prognosis and treatment. Ann Thorac Surg 1991;52:773–8.

29. Deschamps C, Pairolero PC, Trastek VF, et al. Multiple primary lung cancers. J Thorac Cardiovasc Surg 1990;99:769–77.

30. Ferguson MK. Synchronous primary lung cancers. Chest 1993;103:398S–400S.

31. Newman SJ, Hansen HH. Frequency, diagnosis, and treatment of brain metastases in 247 patients with bronchogenic carcinoma. Cancer 1974;33:492–6.

32. Grant FC. Intracranial malignant metastases: their frequency and value of surgery in their treatment. Ann Surg 1926;84:635–46.

33. Cairncross JG, Kim JH, Posner JB. Radiation therapy for brain metastases. Ann Neurol 1980;7:529–41.

34. Mandell L, Hilaris B, Sullivan M, et al. The treatment of single brain metastasis from non-oat cell lung carcinoma: surgery and radiation versus radiation therapy alone. Cancer 1986;58:641–9.

35. Patchell RA, Cirrincione C, Thaler HT, et al. Single brain metastases: surgery plus radiation or radiation alone. Neurology 1986;36:447–53.

36. Patchell RA, Tibbs PA, Walsh JW, et al. A randomized trial of surgery in the treatment of single metastases to the brain. N Engl J Med 1990;322:494–500.

37. Noordijk EM, Vecht CJ, Haazma-Reiche H, et al. The choice of treatment of single brain metastasis should be based on extracranial tumor activity and age. Int J Radiat Oncol Biol Phys 1994;29:711–7.

38. Magilligan DJ, Rogers JS, Knighton RS, et al. Pulmonary neoplasm with solitary cerebral metastasis: results of combined excision. J Thorac Cardiovasc Surg 1976;72(5):690–8.

39. Magilligan DJ, Duvernoy C, Malik G, et al. Surgical approach to lung cancer with solitary cerebral metastasis: twenty-five years' experience. Ann Thorac Surg 1986;42(4):360–4.

40. Read RC, Boop WC, Yoder G, et al. Management of nonsmall cell lung carcinoma with solitary brain metastasis. J Thorac Cardiovasc Surg 1989;98:884–90.

41. Saitoh Y, Fujisawa T, Shiba M, et al. Prognostic factors in surgical treatment of solitary brain metastasis after resection of non-small-cell lung cancer. Lung Cancer 1999;24(2):99–106.

42. Burt M, Wronski M, Arbit E, et al. Resection of brain metastases from non-small-cell lung carcinoma. J Thorac Cardiovasc Surg 1992;103:399–410.

43. Wronski M, Arbit E, Burt M, et al. Survival after surgical treatment of brain metastases from lung cancer: a follow-up study of 231 patients treated between 1976 and 1991. J Neurosurg 1995;83:605–16.

44. Collaud S, Stahel R, Inci I, et al. Survival of patient treated surgically for synchronous single-organ metastatic NSCLC and advanced pathologic TN stage. Lung Cancer 2012;78:234–8.

45. Griffioen GH, Toguri D, Dahele M, et al. Radical treatment of synchronous oligometastatic non-small cell lung carcinoma (NSCLC): patient outcomes and prognostic factors. Lung Cancer 2012;82:95–102.

46. Marabella P, Takita H. Adenocarcinoma of the lung: clinicopathological study. J Surg Oncol 1975;7:205–12.

47. Ettinghausen SE, Burt ME. Prospective evaluation of unilateral adrenal masses in patients with operable non-small cell lung cancer. J Clin Oncol 1991;9(8):1462–6.

48. Beitler AL, Urschel JD, Velagapudi SR, et al. Surgical management of adrenal metastases from lung cancer. J Surg Oncol 1998;69:54–7.

49. Luketich JD, Burt ME. Does resection of adrenal metastases from non-small cell lung cancer improve survival? Ann Thorac Surg 1996;62:1614–6.

50. Downey RJ, Ng KK, Kris MG, et al. A phase II trial of chemotherapy and surgery for non-small cell lung cancer patients with a synchronous solitary metastasis. Lung Cancer 2002;38(2):193–7.

Surgery for Small Cell Lung Cancer

Alberto de Hoyos, MD, Malcolm M. DeCamp, MD*

KEYWORDS

- Small cell lung cancer • Early-stage small cell lung cancer • Lobectomy • Lung resection

KEY POINTS

- Evidence-based guidelines recommend that patients with newly diagnosed SCLC undergo a complete medical history and physical examination, a pathologic review of biopsy specimens, laboratory studies, imaging studies, and if appropriate, mediastinal nodal staging.
- Surgery can be offered to selected patients with early-stage SCLC as part of a multimodality treatment plan.
- With adequate patient selection, rigorous preoperative staging, and combined multimodality therapy, high rates of local control and satisfying long-term outcomes similar to equivalent-stage NSCLC can be achieved.

The American Cancer Society estimated that 222,500 new cases of lung cancer occurred in the United States in 2010.[1] Of these, small cell lung cancer (SCLC) accounted for 14% or 30,000 of these. More than 90% of these patients will die of their disease. The incidence of SCLC has decreased from 25% of all lung cancers in 1993 to approximately 10% to 14% in 2012.[2,3] SCLC is distinct from non–small cell lung cancer (NSCLC) both biologically and clinically. SCLC is also distinguished from NSCLC by its rapid doubling time and early development of widespread intrathoracic lymph node and distant metastases. Small cell carcinoma is exceedingly rare in nonsmokers, and is more common in men. The percentage of women with SCLC has been rising steadily since the 1970s, likely due to trends in smoking behavior. The average age at diagnosis is 65 to 70 years and it is the variety of lung cancer most commonly associated with paraneoplastic syndromes. Although it is the lung cancer most sensitive to chemotherapy and thoracic radiotherapy (TRT), SCLC has a generally poor prognosis.

Approximately two-thirds of patients presenting with SCLC have clinical evidence of hematogenous metastases (M1) or extensive stage (ES) disease, and chemotherapy is the standard of care. Of the remaining one-third of patients with limited-stage (LS) disease, most have clinical evidence of extensive nodal involvement in the hilar (N1), mediastinal (N2-3), or supraclavicular regions (N3). For this reason, surgical resection is seldom offered in LS-SCLC and instead, 4 to 6 cycles of systemic chemotherapy, with concurrent or sequential TRT, has been typically accepted as the cornerstone of therapy. If a complete remission is achieved, prophylactic cranial irradiation (PCI) improves both overall survival and the incidence of brain metastases. Only 4% to 12% of patients with SCLC have very early stage (VES) disease localized to the lung in the form of a solitary pulmonary nodule (T1-2, N0, M0).[4]

We should no longer equate every diagnosis of SCLC with inoperability. The immortalization of old randomized trials demonstrating lack of benefit of surgery carried out in an era using outdated staging tools and methodology and less effective

The authors have nothing to disclose.

Division of Thoracic Surgery, Northwestern Memorial Hospital, Northwestern University Feinberg School of Medicine, 676 North Saint Clair Street, Suite 650, Chicago, IL 60611, USA

* Corresponding author.

E-mail address: mdecamp@nmh.org

Thorac Surg Clin 24 (2014) 399–409

http://dx.doi.org/10.1016/j.thorsurg.2014.07.005

drugs has no validity in the present era and should not influence the current management of patients diagnosed with VES-SCLC. Unfortunately, the National Cancer Institute (NCI) Web site attributes a 1A level of evidence to a trial by the Lung Cancer Study Group performed 20 years ago to make recommendations regarding the role of surgery in LS-SCLC (http://www.cancer.gov/cancertopics/pdq/treatment/small-cell lung/healthprofessional/Page5#Section_110). Moreover, the Web site fails to mention more recent prospective trials or larger studies derived from national data bases that show a benefit of surgery in well-selected patients with SCLC. Continuously over the past several years, data have been gathering in support of surgery for early-stage SCLC. Sadly a pessimistic view about the prognosis of all patients with SCLC prevails. Surgery is often not even addressed in review publications.[5] The American College of Surgeons Oncology Group has proposed a prospective trial to verify the role of surgery plus adjuvant chemotherapy for early-stage (IA-IB) SCLC. This trial will include patients who either are found after resection to have early stage or who have biopsy-proven SCLC. The primary end points will be 3-year survival and recurrence patterns.

Although there are no recent randomized trials or meta-analyses supporting the role of surgery in selected early-stage SCLC, with adequate patient selection (good performance status), rigorous preoperative staging (T1-2, N2-3 disease excluded, M0) and combined multimodality therapy (surgery, chemotherapy ± TRT, and PCI), high rates of local control and satisfying long-term outcomes similar to equivalent-stage NSCLC can be achieved. The most current evidence is derived from small prospective or retrospective studies and analysis of large data bases (levels II–IV evidence).

STAGING OF SCLC

For more than 50 years, SCLC has been staged differently from NSCLC. Because most patients with SCLC present with advanced, metastatic disease, the TNM staging system was thought to be clinically irrelevant and the Veterans Administration Lung Cancer Study Group (VALSG) proposed a simplified staging system for use in their randomized clinical trials and focused on the importance of radiation therapy for local control.[6] This dichotomous system divided SCLC into 2 subgroups termed "limited-stage" (LS) and "extensive stage " (ES). The VALSG system defined LS disease as (1) disease confined to one hemithorax, although local extension may be present; (2) no extrathoracic metastases except

for ipsilateral supraclavicular lymph nodes; and (3) primary tumor and regional lymph nodes that can be encompassed adequately in a safe radiation portal. Tumors with ipsilateral pleural effusion not proven malignant, left recurrent laryngeal nerve involvement, or superior vena cava involvement were still included. ES disease was defined as disease that cannot be classified as LS disease, including malignant pleural or pericardial effusions, contralateral hilar or supraclavicular lymph nodes, and hematogenous metastases. In 1989, the International Association for the Study of Lung Cancer (IASLC) modified the VALSG staging including all nonmetastatic patients in the LS group. The consensus report recommended that LS should be expanded to include patients with contralateral hilar, ipsilateral and contralateral mediastinal, and ipsilateral and contralateral supraclavicular node involvement as well as those with ipsilateral pleural effusions, both positive and negative on cytologic examination. This conclusion was based on the observation that the prognosis of patients with contralateral adenopathy and ipsilateral pleural effusions was superior to those with distant metastases and more closely parallel to that of those with LS disease. In practice, most physicians and clinical trials blend the VALSG and the IASLC criteria by considering contralateral mediastinal and ipsilateral supraclavicular lymph node involvement to be LS. Determining the classification of contralateral supraclavicular or hilar node involvement remained controversial, with treatment usually determined individually based on the ability to include these regions in a safe radiation portal.

Because the TNM staging system requires accurate mediastinal lymph node sampling (either by mediastinoscopy or endobronchial ultrasound) and pathologic confirmation at the time of surgery, and most patients with SCLC seldom present at a stage for which surgery is appropriate (2%–6%), the TNM system has not been routinely applied to SCLC. However, in small surgical series of patients with SCLC, the TNM staging system can identify subgroups of patients with distinct prognoses from within the broad definition of LS.

In the 2007 proposal of the seventh edition of the IASLC staging classification system, it was recommended that the TNM system be applied to SCLC to stratify patients with LS disease.[7,8] This was formally adopted in 2010. The recommendation was based on a prognostic analysis of 12,620 patients with SCLC in the IASLC database, 8088 of whom had TNM staging available. Mediastinal lymph node metastases can be found in up to 50% of patients with clinical N1 disease.[9,10] These data emphasize the importance of aggressively staging the mediastinum in these patients preoperatively and not relying solely on imaging to render therapeutic decisions. Analysis of the data in 349 surgically treated patients with SCLC (2.8%) showed significantly worse survival for patients with LS disease and mediastinal lymph node involvement (N2; Stage III) than for those with no lymph node involvement (Stage I, N0) or with N1 lymph node involvement (Stage II, N1). The 5-year survival rates were 48%, 39%, and 15% for stage I, II, and III, respectively.[8] Corresponding 5-year survival rates for pathologic stage IA, IB, IIA, IIB, IIIA, and IIIB were 56%, 57%, 38%, 40%, 12%, and 0%, respectively.

It is likely that patients with T1-2, N0-1, M0 tumors (stage IA, IB, IIA, IIB) are the same as those previously classified by the University of Toronto Lung Group as "very limited" stage, a subgroup within the LS category and that can benefit from surgical resection as demonstrated by several studies.[11] For the 2014 update, the National comprehensive Cancer Network (NCCN) panel adopted a combined approach for staging SCLC using both the American Joint Committee on Cancer (AJCC) TNM staging system and the older VALSG scheme. The NCCN and American College of Chest Physicians (ACCP) guidelines define LS disease as stages I to III (T any, N any, M0) that can be safely treated with definitive radiation therapy; however, LS excludes T3-4 status due to multiple lung nodules or tumor/nodal volume too large to be encompassed in a tolerable radiation plan. ES disease SCLC is now defined as stage IV (T any, N any, M1a/b), or T3-4 due to multiple lung nodules or tumor/nodal volume too large to be encompassed in a tolerable radiation plan. LS-SCLC can be divided into 4 groups (LS-0, LS-I, LS-II, and LS-III) according to the level of lymph nodes that are positive. As with NSCLC, prognosis is heavily influenced by the presence and location of nodal metastasis.

PATTERNS OF FAILURE IN TREATED SCLC

Before the introduction of effective systemic chemotherapy, median survival for patients with LS and ES were 12 weeks and 5 weeks, respectively.[12–14] Many studies have demonstrated that chemotherapy significantly improves survival when compared with surgery or TRT alone, and modern combination chemotherapy with cisplatinum-etoposide (EP) is the mainstay of therapy for all patients with SCLC. Contemporary median survival for LS disease is 23 months, with a 5-year survival rate of 12% to 17%. For ES disease, median survival is 7 to 12 months but with a 5-year survival of only

2%.[15] Although the combination of chemotherapy plus TRT improves local control and survival in patients with LS versus single-modality treatment, local recurrence rates in these patients are between 35% and 70% despite initial response. Up to 75% of these patients will have residual disease in the specimen if resection is performed.[16,17] This high local failure rate has led to reconsideration of the role of surgery to eradicate the primary tumor and to obtain and improve local control.

The influence of surgery on local recurrence rates and the site of recurrence were analyzed by Elliot and colleagues[18] by correlating autopsy findings with previous treatment and clinical parameters in 537 patients with SCLC. The first site of recurrence in patients with LS-SCLC who achieve complete remission was the primary tumor site followed by hilar/mediastinal lymph nodes. Only 31% of patients who underwent surgery had residual primary tumor, whereas 92% of patients with LS-SCLC who had undergone mediastinoscopy but were treated without surgery had residual disease at the primary site. A report from Eberhardt and colleagues[19] demonstrated 100% local/regional control after complete surgical resection (R0) following induction chemotherapy-TRT for LS-SCLC with a 5-year survival rate of 63%. However, 36% of patients undergoing R0 resection eventually developed distant recurrence. In a study from the University of Toronto, there were 2 comparable groups of patients who underwent induction chemotherapy followed by adjuvant TRT with or without surgical resection. The rate of local recurrences were 9% and 21% in the surgery and radiotherapy arms, respectively, with better survival in the surgical arm (P<.05).[20] Although there are no randomized controlled trials comparing modern chemotherapy-TRT protocols to chemotherapy-TRT with surgery, the impact of surgical therapy on local control seems to be evident and needs to be considered in selected patients with early-stage SCLC.

EVIDENCE SUPPORTING SURGERY FOR SCLC
Prospective Randomized Trials

In 1983, the Lung Cancer Study Group initiated an important prospective randomized trial in which patients with LS-SCLC treated with induction chemotherapy were randomized either to undergo resection or to receive radiotherapy; results of this trial were published in 1994.[21] More than 300 patients were initially treated with 5 cycles of chemotherapy. An objective response was identified in 217 patients and 146 were then randomized to either thoracotomy followed by TRT or TRT alone. All patients subsequently underwent PCI. Median survival was 15.4 months in the trimodality arm (n = 70) and 18.6 months in the chemotherapy + TRT arm (n = 76). No improvement in survival was identified with the addition of surgery to induction chemotherapy and adjuvant TRT. Conclusions are limited, because in the surgical arm, only 77% (n = 54) of patients underwent complete resection. Second, the response rate to chemotherapy was only 65% and neither platinum-based chemotherapy nor concurrent chemoradiotherapy was used. Third, computed tomography/positron emission tomography (CT/PET) was not available at the time and mediastinoscopy was not routinely performed, limiting the ability to identify patients with possible metastatic disease. Fourth, only 19% of all enrolled patients and 41% (29/70) of the surgery patients had clinical stage I disease, the group that is considered most suitable for surgery. Finally, patients with peripheral lung nodules, assumed to be T1, N0 that might be the best candidates for surgery, were specifically excluded in this study.

In the 20 years since this study, no new randomized trials have been conducted; however, this article continues to be cited as level I evidence to discourage the use of surgical resection in SCLC despite all its limitations. New powerful diagnostic tools, such as spiral computed tomography (CT), PET along with mediastinoscopy, endobronchial ultrasound, and the application of the TNM staging system to SCLC now allow for very limited disease to be readily identified as a distinct subset and to be adequately staged preoperatively. In addition, the availability of more effective, multiagent, platinum-based chemotherapeutic regimens introduced in the 1980s and the realization that TRT often fails to provide durable local control, have prompted a reevaluation of the role of surgery in the multimodal approach for a selected group of patients with early-stage SCLC.

Prospective Nonrandomized Trials

In the 1980s, single-institution pilot studies evaluating induction chemotherapy followed by surgical resection for LS-SCLC demonstrated promising 5-year survival rates.[20,22] A prospective study of adjuvant surgical resection after chemotherapy for LS-SCLC demonstrated a 5-year survival of 36%. Patients with pathologic stage I disease had significantly longer survival times than patients with higher-stage disease, leading the investigators to recommend resection only for patients with documented absence of nodal metastases during the preoperative staging.[20] This trial also demonstrated no survival

difference between patients treated with chemotherapy before the operation and those undergoing an initial operation followed by adjuvant chemotherapy. Projected 5-year survival for patients with pathologic stage I was 51% and significantly better than for stage II (28%) or III (19%).[23] They also postulated local relapse or failure to respond to chemotherapy due to the presence of a mixture of NSCLC and SCLC.[24]

Eberhardt and colleagues[19] reported a prospective trial of induction chemotherapy or chemotherapy + TRT followed by surgical resection in patients with LS-SCLC. This trial excluded patients with T1N0 or positive supraclavicular nodes. Forty-six patients were staged according to the TNM system based on imaging and mediastinoscopy and divided into 2 groups. Group I consisted of 8 patients with stage IB/IIA and received 4 cycles of EP. Group II consisted of 22 patients with stage IIB/IIIA and received 3 cycles of EP followed by a fourth cycle of EP plus concurrent hyperfractionated TRT to a total dose of 45 Gy. After completion of induction therapy and repeat mediastinoscopy, patients were eligible for surgical resection. The study also included 16 patients with stage IIIB who received EP plus TRT to a total dose of 50 to 60 Gy. Of the 32 patients assigned to surgical resection, 23 had a complete resection. The actuarial 5-year and 10-year overall survival rates for all patients were 39% and 35%, respectively, whereas the 5-year and 10-year survival rates for patients with initial disease involvement of the mediastinum (T3 or N2, stage IIB/IIIA) were 44% and 41%, respectively.[25] The survival rate for the 8 patients with stage IB/IIA was not reported. Five-year survival for R0 patients was 63% and no differences were observed among patients with pathologic complete response and those with residual viable tumor but completely resected. Up to 34% of the patients undergoing trimodality therapy had a complete pathologic response with no tumor in the specimen, similar to what is seen in patients with NSCLC.[26] Nakamura and colleagues[27] also observed that pathologic nodal status and response to induction chemotherapy were predictors of survival. Downstaging after induction chemotherapy conferred a survival advantage. Survival after lobectomy or bilobectomy was superior then after pneumonectomy.

Tsuchiya and colleagues[10] reported the results of a prospective phase II trial of adjuvant EP chemotherapy after initial surgical resection for stage I to IIIA SCLC. None of the patients received TRT or PCI. The overall 5-year survival rate was 57% for the entire group, 66% for stage I, 56%

for stage II, 13% for stage III, and 73% in the subset of patients with pathologic stage IA disease. There was no difference between stage IA and IB. These survival figures are equivalent to survival rates in patients with equivalent stage NSCLC. The overall local relapse rate was 10%, and varied from 4% in patients with pathologic stage IA to 22% in stage IIIA. In contrast, the distant failure rate was 36% and ranged from 26% in the pathologic stage IA group to 50% in stage IIIA. This study has delineated not only the efficacy of surgery for improved local control but the necessity of PCI even in VES patients after complete surgical resection.

The Japan Lung Cancer Registry Study demonstrated a 5-year survival rate of 52.6% for surgically resected patients with SCLC, which is comparable to that for patients with squamous (59.1%), large cell (53.3%), and adenosquamous cell carcinoma (50.8%).[28,29] In patients with stage I and II, the addition of chemotherapy resulted in better survival then surgery alone. In addition, the 5-year survival rate in patients who received 4 or more cycles of chemotherapy was 80%, as compared with 46% in patients treated with 1 to 3 cycles.[30] In this study, the survival rate was determined by the T and N, with survival rates better for T1 versus T2 versus T3 and N0-1 better than N2.

Fujimori and coworkers[31] reported the results of a prospective phase II trial of induction chemotherapy (EP + doxorubicin) followed by surgical resection in patients with stage I to IIIA SCLC. Patients with clinical stage I and II disease showed a 3-year survival rate of 73%, and even patients with stage IIIA achieved survival of 43%.

Karrer and Ulsperger[32] reported a prospective trial of 183 consecutive patients who underwent complete resection for T1-2N0M0 SCLC. Following resection, the patients underwent adjuvant chemotherapy and PCI. A 4-year survival rate of 63% was reported for patients with pathologic T1-2N0M0 disease and 37% for patients who were upgraded to N2 disease following resection. Patients who had an R0 resection also had a better 3-year survival (44%) than patients who had an R1-2 resection (19%).

Institutional Retrospective Reviews

Several retrospective reviews support surgical resection to improve the outcome of patients with early-stage SCLC. Interpretation of these results is limited by the selection bias inherit in retrospective reviews and by the variable use of chemotherapy and radiotherapy in these studies. In most series, survival rates declined significantly in patients with more advanced disease, leading

to the general recommendation that surgery should be considered in those with stage I or II disease only.

In 1982, Shields and colleagues[33] reported the experience of the Veterans Administration Surgical Oncology Group in 132 patients who underwent resection followed by adjuvant therapy and concluded that surgical resection could be applied in patients with T1-2N0 SCLC but contraindicated in any other category. The overall 5-year survival rate was 23% for the entire cohort, 60% for patients with T1N0M0.

Bedazio and colleagues[34] published a retrospective matched-pair study of 134 patients treated with surgery followed by adjuvant chemotherapy versus nonsurgical management in LS-SCLC. Seventy-six patients with stage I-IIIA and good performance status were treated by surgery + chemotherapy. Median survival for patients treated with and without surgery was 22 and 11 months, respectively, whereas the 5-year survival was 27% and 4%. Subset analysis confirmed significantly longer survival with surgery in all T and N categories except for N2 disease. Local relapse occurred in 15% and 55% of patients treated with and without surgery, respectively, whereas the distant relapse probabilities were similar in both groups (36% and 40% respectively).

Brock and colleagues[35] examined their results on 82 patients who underwent resection with curative intent. Of these patients, 41 underwent adjuvant chemotherapy with a 5-year survival of 68% in patients treated with platinum-based chemotherapy compared with 32% in those treated with a nonplatinum regimen. For the subset of patients with stage I disease treated with platinum-based and nonplatinum-based chemotherapy, the 5-year survival rates were 86% and 42%, respectively. This study showed an impressive 5-year survival rate for patients with stage I SCLC treated with complete resection followed by adjuvant chemotherapy without TRT and demonstrated the superiority of platinum regimens.

National Cancer Database Reviews

Because of the low incidence of N0-1 SCLC, analyses of national cancer databases have been used to help define the role of surgery in larger populations with early stage SCLC. Several of these are summarized in **Table 1**. Rostad and colleagues[36] retrospectively reviewed the National Cancer Registry of Norway and examined data from 697 patients with LS-SCLC. A total of 180 patients were deemed to have stage I disease at presentation, with 111 patients believed to be potentially resectable but who received

Table 1
Surgery for early-stage small cell lung cancer

Primary Author, Publication Year	Database	Limited-Stage Patients	T1-2 Patients (%)	cStage I Patients	cStage II Patients	No. Resected (%)	Median Survival in Months	% 5-y Survival
Schreiber et al,[38] 2010	SEER	14,179	2382 (17)	NR	NR	863 (36)	S+ 28 S− 13 Lobe 65, SLR 25	S+ 53 S− 32
Yu et al,[37] 2010	SEER	NR	NR	1560	0	389 (25)	NR	49[a]
Varlotto et al,[40] 2011	SEER	NR	NR	1690	529	574 (26)	Lobe 50 SLR 30 S− 20	47[a]
Weksler et al,[39] 2012	SEER	NR	NR	2688	880	895 (25)	S+ 34 S− 16	NR
Gaspar et al,[41] 2012	NCDB	25,386	NR	NR	NR	1395 (5)	S+ 31 S− 15 pStage I-II 37	NR

Abbreviations: cStage, clinical stage; Lobe, lobectomy; NCDB, National Cancer Data Base; NR, not reported; pStage, pathologic stage; SEER, Surveillance, Epidemiology and End Results; SLR, sublobar resection; S+, had surgical resection; S−, no surgical resection.
[a] Survival following lobectomy.

chemotherapy or TRT, whereas the remaining 38 underwent resection as part of multimodality therapy. The 5-year survival rate was 45% with surgery and 11% with conventional treatment. The investigators concluded that more patients should have been offered surgical resection.

Several investigators have published retrospective analyses of the Surveillance, Epidemiology, and End Results (SEER) database sponsored by NCI. SEER has been used to track cancer incidence and survival rates since 1973. The SEER database covers approximately 28% of the United States, representative of the diversity of urban, suburban, and rural communities and captures 98% of all cancer cases within the surveyed geographic areas. SEER provides robust information about surgery and TRT but does not provide data on chemotherapy, performance status, or surgical margin status. Yu and colleagues[37] examined SEER and identified 1560 patients with stage I SCLC, of whom 389 underwent resection (25%). Most (63%) underwent lobectomy (n = 247) or pneumonectomy (n = 10), whereas 38 received adjuvant TRT. The 5-year survival rates for patients with resected stage I with and without adjuvant TRT were 57% and 50%, respectively (P = .92). No improvement in cancer-specific death was identified with the addition of adjuvant TRT in

stage I SCLC, similar to what is observed in NSCLC.

Schreiber and colleagues[38] analyzed 14,179 patients in the SEER database with localized (T1-2NxM0) or regional SCLC (T3-4NxM0 or T1-4N1-2M0). A total of 863 patients (6%) underwent resection by lobectomy (60%), pneumonectomy (8%), or sublobar resection (32%). Most patients undergoing lobectomy also received TRT. Of the patients with localized disease who underwent resection, 45% were alive at 5 years, compared with only 14% of the patients with localized disease treated with nonoperative therapy (P<.001). Patients classified as having regional disease who underwent surgery showed a 5-year survival rate of 26% compared with 9% of those treated with conventional therapy (P<.001). A subgroup analysis of the patients who received adjuvant TRT demonstrated that patients with N0-1 disease did not benefit from radiation compared with surgery alone, whereas significant improvement in survival was seen in patients with N2 disease treated with TRT. Furthermore, survival was significantly improved in patients undergoing lobectomy compared with patients undergoing pneumonectomy or sublobar resection. The use of pneumonectomy may imply a more extensive or central tumor, whereas sublobar resection may indicate limited pulmonary function, both of which were associated with decreased long-term survival.

Weksler and colleagues[39] queried the SEER database for patients with stage I (n = 2686 [75%]) or stage II (n = 880 [25%]) SCLC between 1988 and 2007. Of the total 3566 patients, 895 (25%), underwent pulmonary resection: lobectomy (n = 599 [67%]), wedge resection (n = 251 [28%]), pneumonectomy (n = 38 [4%]), or unspecified (n = 7 [1%]). The median survival for patients who underwent resection was 34 months versus 16 months for patients who did not undergo resection (P<.001). Although the best median survival was observed in patients who had lobectomy or pneumonectomy, patients undergoing wedge resection also had better survival than nonsurgical patients treated with TRT alone (28 vs 16 months, P<.001). Resection had a favorable effect on both, stage I and stage II disease. Patients with stage I SCLC had a median survival of 38 months, compared with 16 months following nonsurgical management. Similarly, patients with stage II who had surgical resection had a median survival (25 months) better than patients who did not undergo resection (14 months). In multivariable analysis, having any pulmonary resection decreased the risk of death by 50%.

Another recent analysis of the SEER database by Varlotto and colleagues[40] concluded that surgery is underused in the management of early-stage SCLC and although lobectomy provides optimal local control and leads to superior survival, sublobar resection may also result in superior outcomes than radiotherapy alone. Five-year survival rates for patients undergoing a lobectomy or greater resection was 47% versus 28% and 17% for patients undergoing sublobar resection or TRT respectively (P<.01). This study also demonstrated no benefit of addition of TRT after surgical resection for patients with stage I SCLC.

Gaspar and associates[41] reported the results of their analysis of 68,611 patients with SCLC from the National Cancer Data Base in a joint project with the American College of Surgeons Commission on Cancer and the American Cancer Society. This database contains information on approximately 75% of all newly diagnosed cases of cancer in the United States and includes information regarding chemotherapy. Of the 25,386 patients with LS-SCLC, 1395 (5%) underwent surgical resection either alone (1.7%) or with additional chemotherapy or TRT (3.8%). Surgery decreased the risk of death versus chemotherapy or TRT. In addition, TRT did not improve survival over surgery alone or surgery with chemotherapy in patients with stage I-II disease, but increased survival in patients with stage III disease.

INDICATIONS FOR SURGERY

Evolving from a number of case-series reports and prospective phase II trials, the role of surgery in LS-SCLC has been influenced by several diverse clinical presentations (**Box 1**). For example, (1) surgical resection for LS-SCLC (T1-2, N0) provides the best local control compared with chemotherapy and radiotherapy; (2) small peripheral lesions without any nodal involvement (T1, N0) can occasionally be misdiagnosed as SCLC when they are in fact typical or atypical carcinoid tumors; (3) combined histology tumors may not be completely eradicated by chemotherapy + TRT because the NSCLC component is less sensitive; (4) salvage surgical resection for chemo-resistant localized SCLC or local relapse after an initial response to chemotherapy + TRT may be more effective than current second-line chemotherapy; and (5) surgical resection of a second primary tumor (typically of NSCLC histology) after cure of initial SCLC.

T1-2N0 Disease

Given the high rates of local recurrence after nonsurgical therapy for patients with LS-SCLC (stages IA-IIIB), pulmonary resection warrants strong consideration in well-selected and aggressively

---

Box 1
Indications for surgery in small cell lung cancer

1. Clinical T1-2, N0, M0 disease

   a. Extrathoracic imaging to exclude metastases

   b. Invasive mediastinal staging

2. Solitary pulmonary nodule (SPN) cytologically diagnosed as small cell lung cancer

   a. Small cytologic samples may actually be typical or atypical carcinoid tumors

3. Combined histology tumors

4. Salvage resection if operability and resectability criteria are met for:

   a. Persistent local disease after chemoradiotherapy (possible NSCLC component)

   b. Early local-only relapse (chemo-resistance)

5. New metachronous tumor in small-cell survivor (after complete re-staging)

   a. Likely new NSCLC

staged patients, specifically those with T1-2, N0 disease. The previously reviewed literature supports the role of surgical resection as the optimal modality for local control with the use of platinum-based chemotherapy and PCI for systemic and cerebral control.

If the diagnosis of SCLC is made through a needle biopsy of a pulmonary nodule and LS is suggested on imaging, a thorough investigation to rule out mediastinal lymph node involvement and distant metastases should follow. Workup should include PET imaging, magnetic resonance imaging (MRI) of the brain, and biopsy of mediastinal lymph nodes in all patients. Good surgical candidates with T-1-2N0M0 disease may undergo surgical resection of the tumor (preferably with lobectomy) along with mediastinal lymph node dissection, with the goal of improving local control and possibly overall survival. At surgical exploration, a mediastinal nodal dissection is performed first with frozen section analysis. If nodes are negative or if nodal involvement is found intraoperatively but all disease appears able to be resected with lobectomy or bilobectomy, then it is reasonable to proceed with resection. Pneumonectomy for resection of a central airway tumor or for nodal disease seems likely to be of limited or no benefit. Adjuvant chemotherapy is used, along with PCI in almost all patients, whereas the use of TRT is more controversial but seems to be of benefit only for N2 disease.

Solitary Pulmonary Nodules (SPN)

Because fewer than 5% to 8% of SCLC cases present as solitary pulmonary nodules (SPNs), a diagnosis of SCLC on a fine-needle aspiration biopsy should be viewed with suspicion. Other neuroendocrine tumors, such as carcinoid or large-cell neuroendocrine neoplasm, may be misdiagnosed as SCLC on a small sample. In these cases, a diagnostic thoracoscopic biopsy is recommended after workup to rule out regional or metastatic disease as described previously. If frozen section confirms the possibility of SCLC, the same procedure described previously should be followed.

Combined Histology Tumors

Resected primary SCLC after chemotherapy reportedly contains residual NSCLC histology in 10% to 29% of patients, even in cases that had shown complete response to preoperative chemotherapy.[42,43] Surgical series of neuroendocrine lung tumors revealed that 26% of resected SCLC contained various other histologic types.[44] In studies of induction chemotherapy followed by

adjuvant surgery for pathologically confirmed SCLC, an NSCLC component was found in the resected specimen in 11% to 15% of cases.[45] It is reasonable to offer surgical resection to improve local control if a histologic diagnosis of combined SCLC/NSCLC without nodal involvement is suspected or confirmed. Surgery must be a part of a combined modality approach because surgery alone is not adequate for the SCLC component. An NSCLC component may be responsible for local relapse or the poor response to chemoradiotherapy; therefore, surgery may be offered as a salvage treatment.[24] As residual lesions after systemic chemotherapy using cisplatin/etoposide could contain chemo-resistant SCLC or NSCLC, surgical resection after chemotherapy is justified in such cases.

Salvage Surgery for Initial Treatment Failure or Relapse

When treatment of SCLC is unsuccessful with either persistence of disease or localized recurrence, second-line chemotherapy + TRT is usually ineffective. This has sparked interest in the concept of salvage surgery. Shepherd and colleagues[24] reported on 28 patients who underwent salvage surgery after neoadjuvant chemotherapy ± TRT. The patients were considered to have relapse following complete remission, no response to induction therapy, a partial response followed by local progression while on chemotherapy, or a residual tumor larger than 3 cm. Histopathology revealed SCLC alone in 18 patients, combined tumor in 4, and NSCLC alone in 6. Postsurgical stage was stage I in 4, stage II in 10, and stage III in 14 patients with an overall 5-year survival of 25%.

New Tumors in Survivors of SCLC

In long-term survivors of successfully treated SCLC, there is an increased frequency of second primary tumors, most commonly NSCLC. This was demonstrated by Heyne and colleagues[46] at the MD Anderson Cancer Center when they reviewed 47 patients with more than 2-year survival following successful treatment of SCLC and identified 14 patients with second malignancies. The risk of developing these secondary cancers increases with time from 2% at 2 to 4 years, 12.6% to 14.4% after 10 years, to a 70% actuarial cumulative risk after 5 years. Any patient who develops a second lung lesion after long-term survival following successful treatment of SCLC should not be assumed to have recurrent SCLC. Many times these new malignancies will be NSCLC, which can be potentially cured with surgical resection. These new lesions should be investigated as any new possible lung cancer to rule out regional or metastatic disease. In addition, a needle biopsy may be considered if possible and surgery may be warranted with the potential for long-term cure.[45] Unfortunately, survival is reduced in these patients compared with patients without prior SCLC (median survival 24.5 vs 58.4 months).[47]

CURRENT GUIDELINES AND CONCLUSIONS

Evidence-based guidelines recommend that patients with newly diagnosed SCLC undergo a complete medical history and physical examination, a pathologic review of biopsy specimens (by an experienced pathologist to exclude carcinoid tumors), and laboratory studies, including complete blood count, serum electrolytes, renal and liver function tests, and serum lactate dehydrogenase. Imaging studies should include a CT scan of the chest and upper abdomen, brain imaging (MRI or CT) and PET/CT. PET has been demonstrated to be of significant value in the selection of patients for surgical resection.[48] Additionally, if pleural effusion is present, it should be investigated with thoracentesis and cytology, and if negative or inconclusive, thoracoscopy should be performed. Routine bone marrow examination is not recommended, and should be reserved for patients with peripheral cytopenia and no other evidence of metastatic disease.

If all investigations are negative, suggesting clinical stage I disease, the patient should undergo invasive mediastinal nodal staging (mediastinoscopy, endobronchial ultrasound, transesophageal ultrasound, and/or video-assisted thoracoscopy) to exclude occult nodal disease even if there is no evidence of mediastinal involvement by imaging, because there can be a significant discrepancy between clinical and pathologic staging in SCLC.[8,20] Because of the aggressive nature of SCLC, staging should proceed expeditiously and should not delay the onset of treatment for more than 1 week. The NCCN and ACCP guidelines recommend use of both VALSG and the AJCC TNM system to classify the tumor stage.

The role for surgical resection in the management of early-stage SCLC remains controversial given the lack of level I clinical evidence. Current NCCN Clinical Practice Guidelines in Oncology[49] and the ACCP Evidence-Based Clinical Practice Guidelines[50] recommend surgery only as an initial treatment option in patients with T1-2, N0M0 (stage I) disease confirmed with extrathoracic imaging (grade 2C) and pathologic staging of the mediastinum (grade 1B). Lobectomy with

complete mediastinal lymphadenectomy is considered reasonable. The NCCN panel does not consider sublobar resection appropriate for patients with SCLC. The pneumonectomy rate for SCLC has declined fourfold over the past few decades and is ill-advised.[51,52]

Surgery can be offered to selected higher-stage patients with SCLC as part of a multimodality treatment approach. In proven (N1+) stage II disease, induction concurrent chemoradiotherapy should be given and radical resection should follow with curative intent only if there has been a definite initial response to the induction treatment. In proven cases of stage IIIA disease, if adjuvant surgery is contemplated, a mediastinoscopy should always precede surgical treatment. If mediastinal clearance has not been achieved, surgery is not indicated. Surgical resection in node-positive SCLC must be planned only in the context of clinical trials and after a pathologic response to induction chemoradiation has been confirmed. Data show that patients with clinically staged disease in excess of T1-2, N0 do not benefit from surgery. However, analysis of patients with SCLC within the IASLC database demonstrates that the 1-year and 5-year survival of patients with resected N1 disease are 74% and 33%, respectively.[8]

If postoperative pathologic staging shows no nodal involvement, adjuvant chemotherapy with EP is recommended (Grade 2C). For patients with positive nodes, the NCCN guidelines recommend concurrent chemotherapy + TRT. The role of TRT seems more effective in the presence of N2 disease and there is little evidence that TRT is beneficial for resected patients with isolated N1 disease receiving adjuvant chemotherapy. Prophylactic cranial irradiation is advised to decrease the risk of brain metastases and improve overall survival.[53,54]

Postoperative follow-up is performed at 3-month to 4-month intervals for the first 2 years, every 6 months during years 3 to 5, and then annually. Chest CT scans are performed at every visit. Routine PET/CT scans are not recommended. New pulmonary nodules should initiate workup for a potential new primary tumor because second primary tumors are a frequent occurrence in patients who are cured of SCLC. Smoking cessation should be encouraged for all patients with SCLC because second primary tumors occur less commonly in patients who quit smoking.[55]

We acknowledge that these recommendations represent consensus opinions based on low-level evidence largely consisting of small retrospective reviews, nonrandomized phase II clinical trials, and analyses of large databases. There is a clear need for a randomized controlled investigation to address the role of surgical resection in the multi-modality treatment of early-stage SCLC.

REFERENCES

1. American Cancer Society. Cancer facts & figures 2010. Atlanta (GA): American Cancer Society; 2010. Available at: http://www.cancer.org/cancer/lungcancer-non-smallcell/index.
2. Govindan R, Page N, Morgensztern D, et al. Changing epidemiology of small cell lung cancer in the United States over the last 30 years: analysis of the surveillance, epidemiology and end results database. J Clin Oncol 2006;24:4539–44.
3. Riaz S, Luchtenborg M, Coupland VB, et al. Trends in incidence of small cell lung cancer and all lung cancer. Lung Cancer 2012;75:280–4.
4. Quoix E, Fraser R, Wolkove N, et al. Small cell lung cancer presenting as solitary pulmonary nodule. Cancer 1990;66:577–82.
5. Yip D, Harper P. Predictive and prognostic factors in small cell lung cancer: current status. Lung Cancer 2000;28:173–85.
6. Zelen M. Keynote address on biostatistics and data retrieval. Cancer Chemother Rep 3 1973;4:31–42.
7. Shepherd FA, Crowley J, Van Houtte P, et al. The International Association for the Study of Lung Cancer Staging Project: proposal regarding the clinical staging of small cell lung cancer in the forthcoming (seventh) edition of the tumor, node, metastasis classification for lung cancer. J Thorac Oncol 2007;2:1067–77.
8. Valliers E, Shepherd FA, Crowley J, et al. The IASLC Lung Cancer Staging Project proposals regarding the relevance of TNM in the pathologic staging of small cell lung cancer in the forthcoming (seventh) edition of the TNM classification for lung cancer. J Thorac Oncol 2009;4:1049–59.
9. Inoue M, Nakagawa K, Fujiwara K, et al. Results of preoperative mediastinoscopy for small cell lung cancer. Ann Thorac Surg 2000;70:1620–3.
10. Tsuchiya R, Suzuki K, Ichinose Y, et al. Phase II trial of postoperative adjuvant cisplatin and etoposide in patients with completely resected stage I-IIIa small cell lung cancer: the Japan Clinical Oncology Lung Cancer Study Group (JCOG39101). J Thorac Cardiovasc Surg 2005;129:977–83.
11. Sheperd FA, Ginsberg RJ, Haddad R, et al. Importance of clinical staging in limited small-cell lung cancer: a valuable system to separate prognostic subgroups. The University of Toronto Lung Oncology Group. J Clin Oncol 1993;11:1592–7.
12. Miler AB, Fox W, Tall R. Five-year follow-up of the Medical Research Council comparative trial of surgery and radiotherapy for the primary treatment of small-celled or oat-celled carcinoma of the bronchus. Lancet 1969;2:501–5.
13. Fox W, Scadding JG. Medical Research Council comparative trial of surgery and radiotherapy for primary treatment of small-celled or oat-celled carcinoma of bronchus. Ten year follow-up. Lancet 1973;2:63–5.
14. Mountain C. Clinical biology of small cell lung cancer: relationship to surgical therapy. Semin Oncol 1978;5:272–9.
15. Jackman DM, Johnson BE. Small-cell lung cancer. Lancet 2005;366:1385–96.
16. Passlick B. Can surgery improve local control in small cell lung cancer? Lung Cancer 2001;33:S147–51.
17. Mentzer S, Reilly J, Sugarbaker D. Surgical resection in the management of small cell carcinoma of the lung. Chest 1993;103:349S–51S.
18. Elliott JA, Osterlind K, Hirsch FR, et al. Metastatic patterns in small-cell lung cancer: correlation of autopsy findings with clinical parameters in 537 patients. J Clin Oncol 1987;5:246–54.
19. Eberhardt W, Stamatis G, Stuschke M, et al. Prognostically orientated multimodality treatment including surgery for selected patients of small-cell lung cancer stages IB to IIIB; long term results of a phase II trial. Br J Cancer 1999;81:1206–12.
20. Shepherd F, Ginsberg R, Patterson G, et al. A prospective study of adjuvant surgical resection after chemotherapy for limited small cell lung cancer. A University of Toronto Lung Oncology Group study. J Thorac Cardiovasc Surg 1989;97:177–86.
21. Lad T, Pantadosi S, Thomas P, et al. A prospective randomized trial to determine the benefit of surgical resection of residual disease following response of small cell lung cancer to combination chemotherapy. Chest 1994;106:320S–3S.
22. Baker R, Ettinger D, Ruckdeschel J, et al. The role of surgery in the management of selected patients with small-cell carcinoma of the lung. J Clin Oncol 1987;5:697–702.
23. Shepherd FA, Ginsberg RJ, Feld R, et al. Surgical treatment for limited small-cell lung cancer. The University of Toronto lung oncology group experience. J Thorac Cardiovasc Surg 1991;101:385–93.
24. Shepherd FS, Ginsberg RJ, Patterson GA, et al. Is there ever a role for salvage operations in limited small-cell lung cancer? J Thorac Cardiovasc Surg 1991;101:196–200.
25. Eberhardt W, Korfee S. New approaches for small-cell lung cancer: local treatments. Cancer Control 2003;10:289–96.
26. Eberhardt W, Wilke H, Stamatris G, et al. Preoperative chemotherapy followed by concurrent chemoradiation therapy based on hyperfractionated accelerated radiotherapy and definitive surgery in locally advanced non-small cell lung cancer: mature results of a phase II trial. J Clin Oncol 1998;16:622–34.
27. Nakamura H, Kato Y, Kato H. Outcome of surgery for small cell lung cancer—response to induction

chemotherapy predicts survival. Thorac Cardiovasc Surg 2004;4:206–10.

28. Sawabata N, Miyaoka E, Asamura H, et al, Japanese Joint Committee for Lung Cancer Registration. Japanese Lung Cancer Registry Study of 116663 surgical cases in 2004: demographic and prognosis changes over decade. J Thorac Oncol 2011;6:1229–35.

29. Inoue M, Sawabata N, Okumura M. Surgical intervention for small-cell lung cancer: what is the surgical role? Gen Thorac Cardiovasc Surg 2012;60:401–5.

30. Inoue M, Miyoshi S, Yasumitsu T, et al. Surgical results for small cell lung cancer based on the new TNM staging system. Ann Thorac Surg 2000;70:1615–9.

31. Fujimori K, Yokoyama A, Kurita Y, et al. A pilot phase 2 study of surgical treatment after induction chemotherapy for resectable stage I to IIIA small cell lung cancer. Chest 1997;11:1089–93.

32. Karrer K, Ulsperger E. Surgery for cure followed by chemotherapy in small cell carcinoma of the lung. For the ISC-Lung Cancer Study group. Acta Oncol 1995;34:899–906.

33. Shields TW, Higgins GA Jr, Mathews MJ, et al. Surgical resection in the management of small cell carcinoma of the lung. J Thorac Cardiovasc Surg 1982;84:481–8.

34. Bedazio A, Kurowaski K, Karnicka-Mlodkowska K, et al. A retrospective comparative study of surgery followed by chemotherapy vs non-surgical management in limited disease—small cell lung cancer. Eur J Cardiothorac Surg 2004;26:183–8.

35. Brock M, Hooker C, Syphard J, et al. Surgical resection of limited disease small cell lung cancer in the new era of platinum chemotherapy: its time has come. J Thorac Cardiovasc Surg 2005;129:64–72.

36. Rostad H, Naalsund A, Jacobsen R, et al. Small cell lung cancer in Norway: should more patients have been offered surgical therapy? Eur J Cardiothorac Surg 2004;26:782–6.

37. Yu JB, Decker RH, Detterbeck FC, et al. Surveillance epidemiology and end results evaluation of the role of surgery for stage I small cell lung cancer. J Thorac Oncol 2010;5:215–9.

38. Schreiber D, Rineer J, Weedon J, et al. Survival outcomes with the use of surgery in limited-stage small cell lung cancer: should its role be re-evaluated? Cancer 2010;116:1350–7.

39. Weksler B, Nason K, Shende M, et al. Surgical resection should be considered for stage I and II small cell carcinoma of the lung. Ann Thorac Surg 2012;94:889–94.

40. Varlotto JM, Recht A, Flickinger JC, et al. Lobectomy leads to optimal survival in early-stage small cell lung cancer: a retrospective analysis. J Thorac Cardiovasc Surg 2011;142:538–46.

41. Gaspar L, McNamara E, Greer E, et al. Small-cell lung cancer: prognostic factors and changing treatments over 15 years. Clin Lung Cancer 2012;13:115–22.

42. Prager RL, Foster JM, Hainsworth JM. The feasibility of adjuvant surgery in limited small cell lung cancer: a prospective evaluation. Ann Thorac Surg 1984;38:622–6.

43. Ju MH, Kim HR, Kim JB, et al. Surgical outcomes in small cell lung cancer. Korean J Thorac Cardiovasc Surg 2012;45:40–4.

44. Asamura H, Kameya T, Matsuno Y, et al. Neuroendocrine neoplasms of the lung: a prognostic spectrum. J Clin Oncol 2006;24:70–6.

45. Shepherd F. The role of for surgery in SCLC. In: Movsas B, Langer C, Goldberg M, editors. Controversies in lung cancer. A multidisciplinary approach. New York: Marcel Dekker, Inc; 2002. p. 125–48.

46. Heyne K, Lippman S, Lee J, et al. The incidence of second primary tumors in long term survivors of small cell lung cancer. J Clin Oncol 1992;10:1519–24.

47. Smythe WR, Estrera AL, Swisher SG, et al. Surgical resection of non-small cell carcinoma after treatment for small cell carcinoma. Ann Thorac Surg 2001;71:962–6.

48. Bradley JD, Dehdashti F, Mintum MA, et al. Positron emission tomography in limited-stage small-cell lung cancer: a prospective study. J Clin Oncol 2004;22:3248–54.

49. Available at: http://www.tri-kobe.org/nccn/guideline/lung/english/small.pdf. Accessed July 16, 2014.

50. Available at: http://www.chestnet.org/Guidelines-and-Resources/Guidelines-and-Consensus-Statements/More-Guidelines/Lung-Cancer. Accessed July 16, 2014.

51. Laucchi M, Mussi A, Chella A, et al. Surgery in the management of small cell lung cancer. Eur J Cardiothorac Surg 1997;12:689–93.

52. Rea F, Callegaro D, Favvaretto A, et al. Long term results of surgery and chemotherapy in small cell lung cancer. Eur J Cardiothorac Surg 1998;14:398–402.

53. Shepherd FA, Ginsberg RJ, Evans WK, et al. Reduction in local recurrence and improved survival in surgically treated patients with small cell lung cancer. J Thorac Cardiovasc Surg 1983;86:498–506.

54. Gong L, Wang QI, Zhao L, et al. Factors affecting the risk of brain metastasis in small cell lung cancer with surgery: is prophylactic cranial irradiation necessary for stage I-III disease? Int J Radiat Oncol Biol Phys 2013;85:196–200.

55. Richardson G, Tucker M, Venzon D, et al. Smoking cessation after successful treatment of small-cell lung cancer is associated with fewer smoking related second primary cancers. Ann Intern Med 1993;119:383–90.

Bronchial and Arterial Sleeve Resection After Induction Therapy for Lung Cancer

Antonio D'Andrilli, MD[a],*, Federico Venuta, MD[b,c],
Giulio Maurizi, MD[a], Erino A. Rendina, MD[a,c]

KEYWORDS

- Lung cancer • Sleeve lobectomy • Induction therapy • Chemotherapy • Radiotherapy

KEY POINTS

- There is clear evidence that lobectomy with bronchial and/or vascular reconstruction is oncologically comparable with pneumonectomy.
- Induction therapy may cause additional risks related to the increased difficulty in surgical dissection and to the potential healing impairment of the reconstructed bronchus.
- Although limited data are available in the literature, the few published studies report the possibility of performing even complex bronchovascular reconstructions after neoadjuvant treatment with no increased morbidity and mortality.

INTRODUCTION

Resection and reconstruction of the bronchus, the pulmonary artery (PA), or both associated with lobectomy have proved to be valid therapeutic options for the treatment of centrally located non–small cell lung cancer. These operations are generally indicated to avoid pneumonectomy (PN) in patients with compromised cardiac and/or pulmonary function, but recent experiences have shown that the advantages of sparing lung parenchyma are also evident in patients without cardiopulmonary impairment.

At present, there is clear evidence that lobectomy with bronchial and/or vascular reconstruction is oncologically comparable with PN, with no increased postoperative morbidity, lower mortality, and better quality of life because of lung sparing.[1]

When considering patients with locally advanced non–small cell lung cancer, induction chemotherapy or chemoradiotherapy has become a standardized indication especially in the presence of N2 disease.

However, although the beneficial prognostic effects of neoadjuvant therapy have largely been proved, concern about an increased risk of complications when complex reconstructive procedures are performed after oncologic treatment, has limited the diffusion of such operations within multimodality treatment options. Additional risks may be related to the increased difficulty in surgical dissection caused by diffuse fibrotic reaction, and to the potential healing impairment of the reconstructed bronchus caused by tissue damage and compromised vascularization.

The authors have no disclosures.

[a] Department of Thoracic Surgery, Sant'Andrea Hospital, University LaSapienza, Via di Grottarossa 1035, Rome 00189, Italy; [b] Department of Thoracic Surgery, Policlinico Umberto I, University LaSapienza, Viale del Policlinico, Rome 00161, Italy; [c] Fondazione Lorillard Spencer Cenci – University La Sapienza – Piazzale A. Moro, Rome 5 – 00185, Italy

* Corresponding author. Department of Thoracic Surgery, Sant'Andrea Hospital, Via di Grottarossa 1035, Rome 00189, Italy.

E-mail address: adandrilli@hotmail.com

Data from the literature in the setting of broncho-vascular reconstruction generally refer to patients not undergoing preoperative chemotherapy or chemoradiotherapy, and few data comparing sleeve lobectomy (SL) with PN after induction therapy are available.

INDICATIONS AND PREOPERATIVE EVALUATION

The indication for a sleeve resection in patients with lung cancer is well defined: a tumor located at the origin of a lobar bronchus and/or at the origin of the lobar branches of the PA, but not infiltrating the remaining lobes as far as to require PN. In addition, a sleeve resection may be indicated when N1 nodes infiltrate the bronchus and/or the PA from the outside. This condition can frequently be found in patients with left upper lobe tumors requiring a combined reconstruction of the bronchus and the PA.

It is not always easy to establish the correct indication for a reconstructive procedure before surgery. Computed tomography (CT) with contrast medium is the most used diagnostic tool (**Fig. 1**). Bronchial infiltration can be confirmed more clearly by a preoperative bronchoscopy, and only in a few cases does intraoperative exploration show a tumor infiltration limited to the external surface of the bronchial wall not visible at the endoscopic evaluation.

In contrast, the correct indication for a sleeve resection of the PA may be more difficult to define by the preoperative study. Angiography and magnetic resonance imaging of the blood vessels can provide useful information to assess the pattern of vascular infiltration, but the decision is usually made during surgery.

PA infiltration degree and extension are not always clearly shown at preoperative imaging. Sometimes discrepancies between radiological evidence and intraoperative findings may be responsible for wrong indications, because the preoperative study may overestimate or underestimate the vascular involvement.[2]

Establishing the correct indication generally becomes more complex and controversial after induction therapy. At preoperative CT reevaluation it is usually difficult to distinguish diffuse desmoplastic reaction and fibrosis related to chemotherapy and radiotherapy from residual tumor.

The final decision to perform an SL as an alternative to standard lobectomy or PN is therefore generally taken by the surgeon based on intraoperative findings. Because doubts about the presence of viable tumor in the context of fibrotic scarring tissue may persist, extensive use of intraoperative frozen-section analysis is mandatory in order to choose the most appropriate oncologic operation.

Fiberoptic bronchoscopy is the cornerstone of bronchial evaluation. In the setting of a multimodality treatment including surgery it is important that this examination is performed by one of the operating surgeons, ideally with the possibility of comparing the bronchus status after induction therapy with that observed before the induction therapy. Careful evaluation of the bronchial motion can provide useful information on the state of tissues outside the bronchus: stiffness of the bronchial wall may indicate peribronchial tumor infiltration. Endobronchial ultrasonography has improved the accuracy of bronchoscopic evaluation in recent years.

In patients undergoing induction treatment, endobronchial tumor growth is a frequent finding producing partial or complete airway obstruction. This condition may be responsible for a rapid respiratory and general status deterioration. Also the accuracy of staging may be limited because of the postobstructive lung atelectasis.

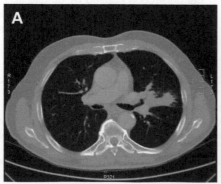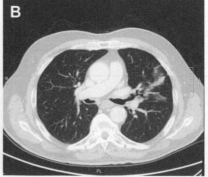

Fig. 1. CT scan images showing a left upper lobe lung cancer infiltrating the bronchus and the PA before (*A*) and after (*B*) induction treatment. The tumor was radically resected by a bronchovascular sleeve resection.

In such clinical situations, neodymium:yttrium-aluminum-garnet laser restoration of an adequate bronchial lumen before induction therapy has proved effective in minimizing the complications related to atelectasis, in improving patient tolerance to induction regimens, and in allowing correct tumor staging.[3]

It is still a matter of debate whether, in cases of viable tumor in the main bronchus at presentation that is no longer visible after neoadjuvant therapy, a parenchyma-sparing operation should be considered instead of a PN.

The primary oncologic goal in every case is the complete resection of the tumor with free resection margins. Based on this principle the authors' approach is to tailor the extent of resection according to the results of frozen-section analysis. This policy is also justified by the evidence from literature data that PN, especially right PN, is itself a disease, with severe impairment of lung function and quality of life after surgery.[4,5] This intervention should therefore be avoided whenever possible.

Another controversial issue is whether the presence of N1 disease should dictate the indication for a PN, because of the higher risk of tumor cell diffusion through the peribronchial lymphatic vessels in the adjacent macroscopically uninvolved lung districts. There is evidence in the literature, for patients with positive hilar nodes, that SL is related to lower morbidity and mortality and better long-term results than PN.[6–8] These data support the choice of a parenchyma-sparing operation in this setting.

OPERATIVE TECHNIQUE
Dissection Phase

After induction treatment, the dissection of the pulmonary hilum and mediastinum can be difficult and hazardous because the bronchial and vascular structures may be embedded in the desmoplastic reaction and scarring tissue produced by the chemotherapy and radiotherapy. Anatomic and technical considerations in this article mainly refer to upper lobe disease because most surgical procedures are performed for tumors originating in this location, whereas reconstructions for tumors of the lower and middle lobe are rarer.

A crucial step of the operation consists in achieving full control of the proximal portion of the PA. The PA can be isolated on both sides extrapericardially if the infiltration is found only distally near the interlobar fissure. However, in many patients the artery may be involved close to its origin, and therefore the pericardium has to be opened to apply the proximal arterial clamping. The pericardium is generally incised longitudinally behind the phrenic

nerve to confirm that the origin of the PA is free from tumor and to allow its preparation.

On the right side, extrapericardial preparation can be facilitated with the anterior and medial retraction of the superior vena cava (SVC). When proximal infiltration of the artery is close to the pericardial reflection, the PA can be isolated and clamped transpericardially between the SVC and the ascending aorta. The vessel is then encircled by an umbilical tape.

In general, the isolation of the pulmonary veins is less problematic because these vessels are located far from most tumors that are amenable to a sleeve resection. Involvement of the superior pulmonary vein can be found on the left side due to the presence of tumors infiltrating the anterior aspect of the upper lobe bronchus (which is located closely posterior) or the anterior portion of the fissure.

On the right side the superior pulmonary vein can be involved because of tumors infiltrating the fissural portion of the PA, which is located tightly behind the vein.

Full control of the main bronchus can be achieved without significant problems if a sleeve resection is technically feasible.

The core of bronchial and/or PA resection is the dissection in the interlobar fissure. The interlobar fissure is generally approached once complete control of the proximal PA has been achieved. Dissection in this site can be safer after proximal clamping of the artery.

Technical expertise and mature surgical judgment are needed, because it is generally in this step of the operation that the tumor can be judged amenable to a sleeve resection or a PN, or considered unresectable.

Shrinkage of tumor and fibrosclerotic reaction produced as a consequence of induction therapy usually increase the technical complexity of surgical dissection and may pose doubt in the identification of viable tumor at this site. Frozen-section histology should therefore be performed on all suspicious tissue.

However, after chemotherapy or chemoradiotherapy, sleeve resection with reconstructive procedures may also be indicated when indissociable fibrotic tissue with no residual tumor is embedded in the bronchus and/or the PA. In some situations both the upper lobe bronchus and the PA can be encased in fibrotic tissue even without tumor cells at frozen-section analysis. Because lobectomy is technically impossible and PN is the alternative, we think that this is a good indication for a combined bronchovascular reconstruction.

During dissection in the fissural plane, exposure of the arterial branches to the superior segment and to the anterior-basal segment of the lower lobe has to confirm that the vasculature to the lower lobe is free from tumor and can be spared. On the right side, it is also essential to verify the integrity of the arterial branch to the middle lobe, otherwise the middle lobe should be included in the resection.

We prefer to approach the fissure on the left side starting from its posterosuperior end, at the level of the main PA, proceeding with the dissection anteriorly and inferiorly in a subadventitial plane.

On the right side we expose the intrafissural artery behind the middle lobe and to identify the branch for the superior segment of the lower lobe by dissecting from front to back. To avoid extensive parenchymal dissection in the fissure the exposure can be continued posteriorly at the bifurcation between the upper lobe bronchus and the bronchus intermedius. A crotch lymph node is a frequent finding in this location. If cleavable, this lymph node can be elevated away from the bifurcation, allowing exposure of the PA branch to the superior segment of the lower lobe. Once this branch is identified, the posterior portion of the fissure can be completed with a linear stapler. The bronchus intermedius is encircled just distal to the upper lobe take-off and an umbilical tape is placed to aid the airway division at the appropriate site.

RESECTION AND RECONSTRUCTION PHASE

The resection phase begins once the main and distal PA, the bronchus, and both pulmonary veins have been duly prepared. Before starting the dissection it is useful to clamp the previously prepared main PA. Clamping of the proximal PA is performed after systemic heparinization. In the past we used to clamp the inferior pulmonary vein to obtain backflow control when a sleeve resection of the artery was required. We now prefer to clamp the PA distally to the tumor infiltration.

The dose of intravenous heparin represents the only intraoperative management modification adopted by the authors over time. We prefer to administer 1500 to 2000 units (about 20–25 units/kg) instead of the dose between 3000 and 5000 units that was used in the past. Heparin dose has been reduced to prevent postoperative oozing, especially from the lymphadenectomy sites, and has proved effective in avoiding the risk of thrombosis. Heparin is not reversed by protamine after declamping once the vascular reconstruction has been completed.

Although dissection after chemotherapy or chemoradiotherapy can be difficult, resection and reconstruction of the PA and bronchus are not usually different from what is routinely performed in standard cases.

Technical aspects of reconstruction of the PA and the bronchus have been addressed in detail in previous publications[9–11] by the current authors and are briefly reported in this article.

BRONCHIAL RESECTION AND RECONSTRUCTION

After complete preparation of the bronchial structures, the mainstem bronchus is divided just proximal to the upper lobe take-off. Once the bronchus has been sectioned proximally, the definitive decision to proceed with a sleeve resection is made based on macroscopic and microscopic findings. The bronchus is divided distally at the inferior upper lobe take-off. Bronchial cuts must be perpendicular to the long axis of the airway (**Fig. 2**). Microscopic tumor found at a bronchial margin requires additional resection of the involved areas or possibly PN.

Different techniques have been described for bronchial anastomotic reconstruction. The present authors' preference is for the use of interrupted sutures of 4/0 monofilament absorbable material.[9] Sutures are placed circumferentially starting from the junction between the cartilaginous and the membranous parts of the bronchus on the mediastinal side and proceeding toward the lateral side. Sutures are subsequently tied after their placement has been completed. By accurately calibrating distances between sutures it is possible to compensate for even large-caliber discrepancies between the 2 bronchial stumps. This technique prevents torsion of the bronchial axis and gently stretches the circumference of the distal bronchus.

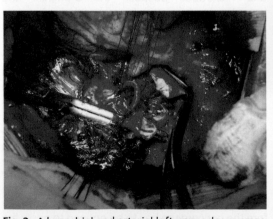

Fig. 2. A bronchial and arterial left upper sleeve resection. The bronchial and clamped arterial stumps are visible before anastomotic reconstruction.

The standardized use of continuous running sutures (complete or partial) has also been reported by other investigators.[12,13]

PA RESECTION AND RECONSTRUCTION

The right and the left PAs can be involved to various extents. In cases of limited, marginal infiltration of the arterial wall, a simple tangential resection with direct suture can be sufficient to achieve a radical exeresis. This technique is generally regarded as a variation of a standard resection and therefore is not considered in this article. In larger defects up to 30% or 40% of the vessel circumference the reconstruction can be performed by a patch (of biological or synthetic material), avoiding a circumferential resection. More extended infiltration requires a sleeve resection and reconstruction by end-to-end anastomosis, or by the interposition of a prosthetic conduit.

Partial Resection and Patch Reconstruction

The patch reconstruction technique can be applied to a variety of conditions. These conditions range from limited infiltration of the origin of segmental arteries to larger resection of the PA involving less than one-half of the vessel circumference. In more extended infiltration a sleeve resection with end-to-end anastomosis or conduit interposition has to be performed.

Various materials have been tested and used for patch reconstruction, including synthetic or biological options, with the latter being preferred because of the higher biocompatibility.

Among the biological materials, the authors recommend the use of the autologous pericardium because it has several advantages: it shows adequate thickness and resistance, it is cost free and available on both sides of the chest, and it has superior biocompatibility compared with the bovine pericardium. Moreover, it provides an amount of tissue that is also sufficient for the repair of large defects, and it does not require a separate surgical procedure for its harvesting. The pericardial tissue usually seems adequate for vascular reconstruction even after induction therapy.

In order to improve the technical features of the autologous pericardium, in the last decade the authors have devised and used an intraoperative method of fixation of the patch by a glutaraldehyde-buffered solution.[14] The glutaraldehyde preservation of the pericardium minimizes its tendency to retract and curl, thus allowing an easier vascular suture. Harvesting of the autologous pericardium is performed anterior to the phrenic nerve, leaving open the pericardial defect. Suturing is done with 5-0 or

6-0 monofilament nonabsorbable material proceeding from top to bottom artery first, and then continuing from bottom to top patch first. In patients also requiring a bronchial anastomosis, the PA patch reconstruction is generally performed first in order to reduce clamping time.

Sleeve Resection and Reconstruction by End-to-end Anastomosis

Sleeve resection of the PA is always required when half or more of the vessel circumference is infiltrated by the tumor. Transection of the artery proximal and distal to the tumor has to ensure regular and even margins to allow subsequent proper placement of sutures (see **Fig. 2**). During the anastomotic suture, regular borders facilitate correction of the caliber discrepancy that is usually found between the 2 vascular stumps after resection. Although the elasticity of the arterial wall may be reduced after induction therapy, caliber discrepancy usually does not present a technical problem.

In patients requiring a concomitant bronchial anastomosis, the PA reconstruction is generally postponed, because exposure of the bronchial stumps is better when the artery is divided. After completion of the bronchial anastomosis the bronchial axis is shortened, thus reducing tension on the vascular anastomosis.

If the distance between vascular stumps appears excessive before reconstruction, a prosthetic conduit interposition is indicated. The anastomosis is performed by running suture using 5-0 or 6-0 monofilament nonabsorbable material (**Fig. 3**).

The mediastinal portion of the anastomosis is performed first, and then the suture is completed in the lateral portion, which is the easiest part of the reconstruction.

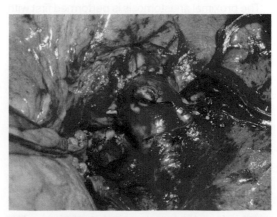

Fig. 3. Completed anastomotic reconstruction of the PA after sleeve resection.

Sleeve Resection and Reconstruction by a Prosthetic Conduit

In some patients after sleeve resection of the PA an excessive distance between the 2 vascular stumps may result. This condition could produce a high tension on the anastomosis. Such technical situations usually occur on the left side in those cases requiring resection of a long segment of the PA without associated bronchial sleeve resection, because the lobar bronchus is not involved. In these cases the vascular reconstruction cannot be performed by a direct end-to-end anastomosis and a prosthetic conduit interposition is required.

Although the need for a vascular conduit is not a frequent condition, various materials and techniques have been proposed for this reconstructive procedure.

The authors have reported the successful use of autologous and bovine pericardium.[15] When the autologous pericardium is used the pericardial leaflet is trimmed to a rectangular shape and wrapped around a chest tube or a syringe of an appropriate diameter and closed longitudinally by a manual or mechanical suture. The epicardial surface is oriented inside the conduit lumen.

An alternative for conduit reconstruction is the pulmonary vein of the resected lobe when the extraparenchymal portion of this vessel is free from tumor.[16] The superior pulmonary vein is sutured proximally by a thoracoabdominal stapler (30 mm) and is ligated distally at the extralobar origin of its branches. The vein is then sectioned proximally and distally between sutures, so that a 1.5-cm to 2.5-cm conduit is obtained. The venous conduit is an ideal autologous prosthesis for PA replacement because it has adequate thickness and structural similarity with the arterial wall.

The use of cryopreserved allograft for PA replacement in conduit reconstruction has been also successfully reported by other investigators.[17]

The proximal anastomosis is performed first with running 5-0 monofilament suture. The distal anastomosis is then performed with the same technique, after the conduit length has been checked.

Care must be taken to avoid lengthening of the reconstructed PA, which may cause kinking of the vessel, impaired blood flow, and ultimately thrombus formation.

COMPLICATIONS AND PERIOPERATIVE MANAGEMENT

A good final outcome in every reconstructive procedure of the bronchus and PA is principally the result of meticulous surgical technique. The preoperative administration of chemotherapy or chemoradiation may theoretically represent an additional risk factor for postoperative complications with a special concern for vasculature and trophism of the bronchial wall.

Technical complications after bronchial reconstruction mainly include anastomotic problems. The occurrence of stenotic complications (minor complications) such as granuloma formation and circumferential scar stenosis is generally not increased after induction therapy and the resolution can usually be achieved by endoscopic procedures.

A theoretic increased risk of anastomotic dehiscence has been reported by many surgeons because tissue damage and fibrotic alteration induced by the induction therapy may be responsible for compromised healing of the reconstructed bronchus.

Based on their long-term experience, the current authors are convinced that protection of the bronchial anastomosis by viable tissue is an effective procedure to minimize the risk of anastomotic dehiscence. The authors' preference is for the intercostal muscle flap, which is easy to prepare, provides excellent vascularization even after neoadjuvant treatment, and perfectly fits the anatomy of the bronchus. This muscle flap may allow preservation of airtightness at the bronchial level even in cases of small anastomotic dehiscence and it has been proved to develop a fine vascular network around the anastomosis after the early postoperative period.[18]

In addition, the occurrence of bronchoarterial fistula, which is a rare but generally catastrophic event, can be prevented by the use of a vascularized flap, especially in patients undergoing combined bronchovascular reconstruction. The muscle interposition between the bronchial and vascular structures in such cases minimizes the risk of PA erosion and consequent fatal bleeding. Even after neoadjuvant therapy the intercostal muscle seems not to be significantly impaired and is adequate for wrapping the reconstructed bronchus. Although some investigators[19] have reported the risk of severe bronchial stenosis caused by the progressive heterotopic calcification of this muscular flap, the present investigators have not observed such a complication.[20]

As an alternative, the use of mediastinal fat pad, pericardial or pleural flap, omentum, or internal mammary artery pedicles has been reported by other investigators, with the general consensus that these techniques may help to reduce the risk of dehiscence.[12,21,22]

However, in the Zurich University Hospital experience, no bronchial anastomotic complication was reported in 25 consecutive patients undergoing bronchial reconstruction after chemotherapy or chemoradiotherapy without viable flap protection.[13]

On the vascular side, an increase of the complication risk caused by induction therapy is generally not reported for PA reconstructive procedures.

The 2 main technical complications after PA reconstruction are bleeding and thrombosis of the reconstructed vessel, which are both considered not to be significantly influenced by the neoadjuvant treatment.

Postoperative bleeding may be related to leakage from the suture line of the anastomotic or patch reconstruction. Because the PA is a low-pressure vessel, oozing may be not identified during surgery, but it can occur later, once lung reexpansion has been completed, because of modification in the PA axis. This modification can distort the suture line and reopen bleeding sites several hours after chest closure. Because the chemotherapy and radiotherapy may reduce the lung parenchyma elasticity, residual lobe reexpansion after induction treatment is sometimes slower than in standard cases. Such phenomena may explain unexpected blood loss beginning in the second or third postoperative day with spontaneous resolution within 24 to 48 hours, as observed by the authors.

Accurate intraoperative checking of the suture line even after lung reinflation may help to reduce the risk of this complication.

Lower lobe reexpansion after PA reconstruction may also promote the occurrence of thrombosis because of kinking and folding over on itself produced by the repositioning of the reconstructed vessel.

In the postoperative period, it is advisable to administer a low-dose anticoagulation therapy (6000–8000 units/d low-weight heparin subcutaneously) for 1 week. This pharmacologic management contributes to reducing the risk of thrombosis.

However, thrombosis represents a rare event if a patch or anastomotic reconstruction is performed. In contrast, higher rates of this complication have been reported after tangential resection with direct suture repair.[23,24]

The postoperative use of systemic steroids (oral or intravenous) in patients undergoing bronchial reconstruction is controversial. The present authors think that the antiedema effect of steroids is beneficial because it reduces secretion retention and atelectasis, it facilitates parenchymal reexpansion, and it minimizes the risk of granuloma formation without increasing the risk of anastomotic dehiscence.[25] Aerosolized steroids (methylprednisolone 5 mg twice a day) are also part of our preoperative (when sleeve resection can be predicted beforehand) and postoperative management. In the authors' experience patients receiving steroidal treatment have shown a reduced need for bronchial aspiration in the postoperative period.

SHORT-TERM AND LONG-TERM RESULTS

There is now evidence from several retrospective studies and meta-analyses that SL represents an adequate therapeutic option for centrally located lung tumors allowing lower morbidity and mortality associated with similar oncologic radicality compared with PN.[1] Parenchyma-sparing operations are also supported by higher survival rates in patients with stage I to II tumors, which is mainly justified by the lower incidence of non–cancer-related deaths.

However, these results are principally from patients not undergoing neoadjuvant therapy, and only limited data are available assessing the role of reconstructive procedures after preoperative chemotherapy or chemoradiotherapy (**Table 1**).

In their initial experience the current authors first reported in 1997 the possibility of performing bronchial and arterial sleeve resection after induction chemotherapy with no mortality, no bronchial and vascular complications, and no local recurrence in the airway. The overall perioperative morbidity rate in a series of 27 patients was similar to that reported in patients undergoing postinduction standard resection in the same period. In addition, 1-year and 4-year survival rates (78% and 39%) did not show significant differences from those reported in the standard resection series (65% and 36%).[26,27]

These results have subsequently been reproduced and further developed by other investigators worldwide, but available data remain limited, with the largest published series including fewer than 50 patients.

In a retrospective study in 2009, Bagan and colleagues[28] reported a comparison between 42 patients undergoing SL after preoperative chemotherapy and 117 patients receiving the same operation without induction therapy over a 22-year period. No significant difference was reported in postoperative morbidity (23.8% vs 24.7%) and mortality (1.7% vs 2.3%). Major anastomotic complications did not occur after chemotherapy, but were observed in 3 patients (2.6%) undergoing surgery alone. The local recurrence rate was 4% in both groups. The 5-year survival rate was higher after induction therapy (74% vs 65.4%), but without a statistically significant difference.

Table 1
Bronchovascular resections after induction therapy. Complications and mortality

Author, Year	Study Period	CHT (n)	CHT-RT (n)	Complications (%)	Mortality (%)	Major Anastomotic Complications (%)	Minor Anastomotic Complications (%)
Rendina et al,[26] 1997	1991–1996	27	—	11	0	0	0
Burfeind et al,[32] 2005	1997–2004	4	15	42	0	5.2	0
Cerfolio,[32] 2007	1998–2006	6	17	26.2[a]	2.4[a]	0	0
Rea et al,[29] 2008	1980–2005	14	10	—	4.5	—	—
Bagan et al,[28] 2009	1984–2005	42	—	23.8	1.7	0	0
Milman et al,[31] 2009	1983–2008	—	21	42.9	0	0	0
Gomez-Caro et al,[17] 2012	2005–2010	—	26	35	0	0	0
Maurizi et al,[33] 2013	1998–2011	39	—	28.2	0	0	2.6

Abbreviations: CHT, chemotherapy; CHT-RT, chemoradiotherapy.
[a] Including patients without induction therapy.

Preoperative irradiation has been identified as an adverse factor for early bronchial anastomotic leak. In particular, the risk of bronchoarterial fistula can be significantly increased, and this complication has been responsible for up to 44% of postoperative mortality following radiotherapy in some series.[29]

In a Japanese[30] study assessing bronchial mucosal blood flow before and after induction therapy, a 30% flow reduction was found after chemoradiation, whereas no significant impairment was observed without induction therapy or after chemotherapy alone. Poor healing of the bronchial stump and increased bronchopleural fistula rate were also reported in patients receiving irradiation.

However, more recent experiences have shown the possibility of achieving satisfactory results even with the use of radiotherapy in addition to preoperative chemotherapy.[17,31]

Gomez-Caro and colleagues[17] analyzed results of bronchial and/or vascular SL, comparing 26 patients receiving induction chemoradiotherapy with 53 patients without induction therapy. There was no difference with respect to complication rate between the patients receiving chemoradiotherapy and the patients not receiving chemoradiotherapy (30% vs 35%). Mortality occurred in only 3 patients of the nonradiochemotherapy group caused by bronchovascular fistula, post-PN pneumonia following PA thrombosis, and acute respiratory distress syndrome. The rate of distant metastasis was similar in both groups and only 1 patient experienced local (mediastinal) recurrence in the induction therapy group. Overall 5-year survival rate was lower after induction therapy (33% vs 69%) as expected because of the more advanced stage tumors included in this group. Vascular reconstruction, upper-left SL, and pathologic N1 disease were independent risk factors for postoperative complications in this study.

Another retrospective study published in 2009 by Milman and colleagues[31] deals with the impact of neoadjuvant chemoradiotherapy on anastomotic complications after sleeve resection. Twenty-one patients underwent parenchyma-sparing operations after different chemoradiotherapeutic (radiation range, 2000–6100 cGy) regimens over 26 years and were compared with 43 patients who received parenchyma-sparing resection alone. The incidence of major complications did not show statistically significant difference: 42.9% in the chemoradiotherapy group, with no anastomosis-related complications, and 46.5% in the surgery-alone group, with 2 anastomotic complications (1 stenosis, 1 bronchovascular fistula). The 90-day postoperative mortalities were also statistically comparable (0% after chemoradiotherapy and 2.7% without induction therapy). Five-year survival rate was 41% in the chemoradiotherapy group compared with 48% in the surgery-alone group ($P = .63$). There were 10% of patients with local recurrence after induction therapy versus 9% of patients without induction therapy ($P = .65$). Eighty percent of patients presenting persistent N2 disease at the time of surgery after induction therapy died within 2 years. This observation prompted the investigators to suggest caution in offering a sleeve resection in this subset of patients.

Burfeind and colleagues[33] analyzed morbidity and mortality data from a series of 19 bronchoplastic procedures after chemoradiotherapy (15) or chemotherapy (4). The overall 30-day early complication rate was 42%, whereas it was 30% in 54 patients who underwent bronchoplasty without preoperative treatment in the study period, but no significant difference was found between the two groups ($P = .6$). The bronchopleural fistula rate was 5.2% in the induction therapy group and 1.3% in the whole study population. Despite the limited bronchial complication rate, an increased need for interventional bronchoscopic procedures was apparent in the surgery-alone group (13% vs 0%). There were 2 (2.7%) 30-day deaths, both in the group not receiving induction therapy.

More recently, the present authors compared results of a group of 39 patients who underwent bronchial and/or arterial SL after chemotherapy with those of 138 patients who received the same operation without induction therapy.[34] The analysis of postoperative complication rates did not show a significant difference (28.2% vs 23.2%; $P = .5$). There was also no significant difference in terms of postoperative mortality (0% vs 0.7%; $P = .5$). The incidence of anastomotic complications (stenosis in all patients) was comparable in the two groups (2.6% vs 3.6%). Mean postoperative hospitalization was 7.8 days after induction therapy and 7.5 days without induction therapy.

When considering pattern of recurrence in studies discussed earlier focusing on SL after induction therapy, it is the usual finding that most patients die because of distant recurrences and that the local recurrence rates are not different between sleeve and standard major resection without neoadjuvant treatment. This finding suggests that SL is effective in locoregional control even in advanced stage tumors as part of multimodality treatment (**Table 2**).

Comparison Between Bronchovascular Reconstructions and PN After Induction Therapy

The postoperative morbidity and mortality risk after induction therapy has often been significantly increased when PN, especially right PN, is performed. The mortality following PN after induction therapy has been reported to be between 14% and 43% in recent large series.[4,35]

In 2013 the authors published the long-term results of their experience comparing SL with PN after induction chemotherapy.[34] A total of 39 patients undergoing bronchial and/or vascular reconstruction associated with lobectomy were analyzed and compared with 39 patients undergoing PN over a 14-year period.

Table 2
Bronchovascular resections after induction therapy. Survival and recurrence rates

Author, Year	CHT (n)	CHT-RT (n)	5-y Survival (%)	Local Recurrence (%)	Distant Recurrence (%)
Rendina et al,[26] 1997	27	—	78 (4-y)	—	48
Bagan et al,[28] 2009	42	—	74	4	—
Milman et al,[31] 2009	—	21	41	10	—
Gomez-Caro et al,[17] 2012	—	26	33	3.8	38
Maurizi et al,[33] 2013	39	—	64	5	15

Because induction radiotherapy was not routinely administered, patients receiving preoperative irradiation were not considered in this study. PA sleeve resection was performed in 18 patients and it was associated with bronchial sleeve resection in 6 of them.

Clinical stage before induction was IIB in 7 patients (6 in the SL group; 1 in the PN group), IIIA in 66 (30 in the SL group; 36 in the PN group), and IIIB in 5 patients (3 in the SL group; 2 in the PN group). The rate of downstaged patients (pathologic complete response and pathologic stage I and II) was 79.5% in the SL group and 53.8% in the PN group ($P = .01$).

Postoperative complications occurred in 28.2% of patients receiving bronchovascular reconstruction and in 33.3% of the PN group, without a statistically significant difference between the two surgical options. Complications related to the reconstructive procedure occurred in 1 patient: a late stenosis of the bronchial anastomosis was observed and it was successfully treated by laser and stenting. Postoperative mortality in the PN group was 2.6%, whereas there was no mortality in the SL group. The difference in postoperative mortality was not significant ($P = .3$). Three-year and 5-year survival rates were 68% and 64% after SL and 59% and 34% in the PN group ($P = .02$).

The tumor recurrence rate was 20.5% in the SL group (locoregional in 2 patients, distant in 6) and 30.8% in the PN group (locoregional in 1 patient, distant in 11), but this difference was not significant. In particular, there was no significant difference between the two groups in locoregional recurrence rate only.

In the study by Bagan and colleagues,[28] the 5-year survival rate in the 42 patients undergoing SL after induction therapy was significantly higher (74%) than that observed in 197 patients receiving postinduction therapy PN (33%; $P = .0006$) in the same period.

Impact on Postoperative Quality of Life

Postoperative quality of life has been advocated as one of the strongest indicators that should influence the decision to perform an SL rather than a PN. Although no specific analysis has been published so far focusing on SL after induction therapy in this setting, several studies indicate that lung parenchyma sparing improves postoperative quality of life, determining a greater cardiopulmonary reserve, less pulmonary edema, and less right ventricular dysfunction caused by a lower pulmonary vascular resistance. In the meta-analysis by Ferguson and Lehman,[36] the quality-adjusted years quoted were 4.37 after SL and

2.48 after PN. Melloul and colleagues[37] analyzed postoperative forced expiratory volume in 1 second (FEV_1) in a retrospective study reporting significantly higher values for patients undergoing SL. In a prospective study by Martin-Ucar and colleagues[38] the reported mean FEV_1 loss after parenchyma-sparing operations was 170 mL (range, 0–500 mL) compared with 600 mL (range, 200–1400 mL) after PN, indicating a significant functional advantage for patients undergoing SL.

ACKNOWLEDGMENTS

The authors thank Dr Marta Silvi for data management and editorial work.

REFERENCES

1. Ma Z, Dong J, Fan J, et al. Does sleeve lobectomy concomitant with or without pulmonary artery reconstruction (double sleeve) have favorable results for non-small cell lung cancer compared with pneumonectomy? A meta-analysis. Eur J Cardiothorac Surg 2007;32:20–8.
2. Ciccone AM, D'Andrilli A, Venuta F, et al. Imaging of tumor infiltration of the pulmonary artery amenable to sleeve resection. J Thorac Cardiovasc Surg 2008;136:229–30.
3. Venuta F, Rendina EA, De Giacomo T, et al. Endoscopic treatment of lung cancer invading the airway before induction chemotherapy and surgical resection. Eur J Cardiothorac Surg 2001;20:464–7.
4. Venuta F, Anile M, Diso D, et al. Operative complications and early mortality after induction therapy for lung cancer. Eur J Cardiothorac Surg 2007;31(4):714–7.
5. Albain KS, Swann RS, Rusch VW, et al. Radiotherapy plus chemotherapy with or without surgical resection for stage III non-small-cell lung cancer: a phase III randomised controlled trial. Lancet 2009;374:379–86.
6. Deslauriers J, Grégoire J, Jacques LF, et al. Sleeve lobectomy versus pneumonectomy for lung cancer: a comparative analysis of survival and sites of recurrence. Ann Thorac Surg 2004;77:1152–6.
7. Kim YT, Kang CH, Sung SW, et al. Local control of disease related to lymph node involvement in non-small cell lung cancer after sleeve lobectomy compared with pneumonectomy. Ann Thorac Surg 2005;79:1153–61.
8. Parissis H, Leotsinidis M, Hughes A, et al. Comparative analysis and outcomes of sleeve resection versus pneumonectomy. Asian Cardiovasc Thorac Ann 2009;17:175–82.
9. Rendina EA, Venuta F, Ciriaco P, et al. Bronchovascular sleeve resection. Technique, perioperative management, prevention of treatment complications. J Thorac Cardiovasc Surg 1993;106:73–9.

10. Venuta F, Ciccone AM, Anile M, et al. Reconstruction of the pulmonary artery for lung cancer: long-term results. J Thorac Cardiovasc Surg 2009; 138(5):1185–91.

11. Ibrahim M, Maurizi G, Venuta F, et al. Reconstruction of the bronchus and pulmonary artery. Thorac Surg Clin 2013;23:337–47.

12. Yldizeli B, Fadel E, Mussot S, et al. Morbidity, mortality and long-term survival after sleeve lobectomy for non-small cell lung cancer. Eur J Cardiothorac Surg 2007;31:95–102.

13. Storelli E, Tutic M, Kestenholz P, et al. Sleeve resections with unprotected bronchial anastomoses are safe even after neoadjuvant therapy. Eur J Cardiothorac Surg 2012;42:77–81.

14. D'Andrilli A, Ibrahim M, Venuta F, et al. Glutaraldehyde preserved autologous pericardium for patch reconstruction of the pulmonary artery and superior vena cava. Ann Thorac Surg 2005;80:357–8.

15. Rendina EA, Venuta F, Degiacomo T, et al. Sleeve resection and prosthetic reconstruction of the pulmonary artery for lung cancer. Ann Thorac Surg 1999;68:995–1002.

16. Cerezo F, Cano JR, Espinosa D, et al. New technique for pulmonary artery reconstruction. Eur J Cardiothorac Surg 2009;36(2):422–3.

17. Gomez-Caro A, Boada M, Reguart N, et al. Sleeve lobectomy after induction chemoradiotherapy. Eur J Cardiothorac Surg 2012;41:1052–8.

18. Rendina EA, Venuta F, Ricci C, et al. Protection and revascularization of bronchial anastomoses by the intercostal pedicle flap. J Thorac Cardiovasc Surg 1994;107:1251–4.

19. Deeb ME, Sterman DH, Shrager JB, et al. Bronchial anastomotic stricture caused by ossification of an intercostals muscle flap. Ann Thorac Surg 2001;71: 1700–2.

20. Ciccone AM, Ibrahim M, D'Andrilli A, et al. Ossification of the intercostals muscle around the bronchial anastomosis does not jeopardize airway patency. Eur J Cardiothorac Surg 2006;29:602–3.

21. D'Andrilli A, Venuta F, Menna C, et al. Extensive resections: pancoast tumors, chest wall resections, en bloc vascular resections. Surg Oncol Clin N Am 2011;20:733–56.

22. D'Andrilli A, Ibrahim M, Andreetti C, et al. Transdiaphragmatic harvesting of the omentum through thoracotomy for bronchial stump reinforcement. Ann Thorac Surg 2009;88(1):212–5.

23. Read RC, Ziomek R, Ranval TJ, et al. Pulmonary artery sleeve resection for abutting left upper lobe lesions. Ann Thorac Surg 1993;55:850–4.

24. Wada H, Okubo K, Hirata T, et al. Evaluation of cases with combined bronchoplasty and pulmonary arterioplasty for the treatment of lung cancer. Lung Cancer 1995;13:113–20.

25. Rendina EA, Venuta F, Ricci C. Effects of low-dose steroids of bronchial healing after sleeve resection. A clinical study. J Thorac Cardiovasc Surg 1992; 104:888–91.

26. Rendina EA, Venuta F, De Giacomo T, et al. Safety and efficacy of bronchovascular reconstruction after induction chemotherapy for lung cancer. J Thorac Surg 1997;114:830–7.

27. Rendina EA, Venuta F, De Giacomo T, et al. Sleeve resection after induction therapy. Thorac Surg Clin 2004;14:191–7.

28. Bagan P, Berna P, Brian E, et al. Induction chemotherapy before sleeve lobectomy for lung cancer: immediate and long-term results. Ann Thorac Surg 2009;88(6):1732–5.

29. Rea F, Marulli G, Schiavon M, et al. A quarter of a century experience with sleeve lobectomy for non-small cell lung cancer. Eur J Cardiothorac Surg 2008;34:488–92.

30. Yamamoto R, Tada H, Kishi A, et al. Effects of preoperative chemotherapy and radiation therapy on human bronchial blood flow. J Thorac Cardiovasc Surg 2000;119:939–45.

31. Milmann S, Kim AW, Warren WH, et al. The incidence of perioperative anastomotic complications after sleeve lobectomy is not increased after neoadjuvant chemoradiotherapy. Ann Thorac Surg 2009;88:945–51.

32. Cerfolio RJ, Bryant AS. Surgical techniques and results for partial or circumferential sleeve resection of the pulmonary artery for patients with non-small cell lung cancer. Ann Thorac Surg 2007;83(6):1971–6.

33. Burfeind WR, D'Amico TA, Toloza EM, et al. Low morbidity and mortality for bronchoplastic procedures with and without induction therapy. Ann Thorac Surg 2005;80:418–22.

34. Maurizi G, D'Andrilli A, Anile M, et al. Sleeve lobectomy compared with pneumonectomy after induction therapy for non-small cell lung cancer. J Thorac Oncol 2013;8:637–43.

35. Daly BD, Fernando HC, Ketchedjian A, et al. Pneumonectomy after high-dose radiation and concurrent chemotherapy for non-small-cell lung cancer. Ann Thorac Surg 2006;82:227–31.

36. Ferguson MK, Lehman AG. Sleeve lobectomy or pneumonectomy: optimal management strategy using decision analysis techniques. Ann Thorac Surg 2003;76(6):1782–8.

37. Melloul E, Egger B, Krueger T, et al. Mortality, complications and loss of pulmonary function after pneumonectomy vs. sleeve lobectomy in patients younger and older than 70 years. Interact Cardiovasc Thorac Surg 2008;7:986–9.

38. Martin-Ucar AE, Chaudhuri N, Edwards JG, et al. Can pneumonectomy for non-small cell lung cancer be avoided? An audit of parenchymal sparing lung surgery. Eur J Cardiothorac Surg 2002;21(4):601–5.

Advanced Lung Cancer
Aggressive Surgical Therapy Vertebral Body Involvement

Mark H. Bilsky, MD[a], Ilya Laufer, MD[a], Evan Matros, MD[b],
Joshua Yamada, MD[c], Valerie W. Rusch, MD[d],*

KEYWORDS

- Lung cancer • Spine involvement • NOMS

KEY POINTS

- The neurologic, oncologic, mechanical, and systemic (NOMS) paradigm provides a dynamic and adaptable decision framework that allows incorporation of evolving treatment options to facilitate the determination of optimal treatment of spinal metastases.
- Stereotactic radiosurgery provides consistent local control in the treatment of non-small cell lung carcinoma (NSCLC) metastases to the spine, whereas conventional external beam radiation therapy often fails to provide long-term local control.
- Patients with spinal cord compression secondary to NSCLC metastases require spinal cord decompression and spinal stabilization.
- SRS provides local control regardless of tumor size and previous radiation, thereby obviating aggressive cytoreductive excision of NSCLC spinal metastases.
- Spinal Instability Neoplastic Score facilitates diagnosis of spinal instability. Patients with spinal instability require intervention for stabilization.

INTRODUCTION

Non-small cell lung carcinoma (NSCLC) presenting with vertebral body or spine involvement is most commonly the result of metastatic disease but can also result from direct extension exemplified by superior sulcus tumors. Discussion on superior sulcus tumors can be found in numerous other places throughout the literature; however, the evaluation and techniques for tumors involving the vertebral body are similar to those discussed in this article. The goals of treatment of metastatic disease to the spine from NSCLC are palliative, with the goals of achieving pain and local-tumor

control, preserving or improving neurologic function, and providing mechanical stability. Traditionally, the principal modalities to treat spine tumors have been open surgery and/or conventional external beam radiation therapy (cEBRT), such as 30 Gy in 10 fractions. However, the past decade has witnessed an explosion of new technologies applied to spine metastases that have significantly improved patient outcomes but also significantly complicated decision making. These new treatment modalities include less invasive surgical approaches and decompressive techniques, including screw-rod instrumentation, percutaneous cement augmentation, and pedicle screw

The authors have nothing to disclose.
[a] Department of Neurosurgery, Memorial Sloan-Kettering Cancer Center, 1275 York Avenue, New York, NY 10065, USA; [b] Plastic Surgery Service, Department of Surgery, Memorial Sloan-Kettering Cancer Center, 1275 York Avenue, New York, NY 10065, USA; [c] Department of Radiation Oncology, Memorial Sloan-Kettering Cancer Center, 1275 York Avenue, New York, NY 10065, USA; [d] Thoracic Surgery Service, Department of Surgery, Memorial Sloan-Kettering Cancer Center, 1275 York Avenue, New York, NY 10065, USA
* Corresponding author.
E-mail address: ruschv@mskcc.org

thoracic.theclinics.com

fixation. The most important advance has been the evolution and integration of stereotactic radiosurgery (SRS), typically as a 24 Gy single fraction or 8 Gy × 3 fractions, used as definitive treatment or as a postoperative adjuvant therapy. The multidisciplinary spine team at Memorial Sloan-Kettering Cancer Center uses a decision framework, NOMS, which incorporates the four fundamental assessments used in decision making: neurologic, oncologic, mechanical instability, and systemic disease. NOMS provides the means of assessing spine metastases that incorporates advances in radiation and medical oncology, interventional radiology, and surgery to optimize patient outcomes.[1]

NOMS DECISION FRAMEWORK FOR SPINE METASTASES

In the NOMS decision framework, the neurologic assessment principally reflects the degree of epidural spinal cord compression (ESCC) based on a validated scoring system using MRI axial T2-weighed images.[2] This scoring system is used to differentiate no or minimal ESCC (0–1) from high-grade spinal ESCC 2–3. Additionally, the neurologic consideration is affected by the presence or absence of myelopathy and/or functional radiculopathy. The oncologic consideration is predicated on the known cytotoxicity and the durability of the response to current treatment modalities including cEBRT, SRS, chemotherapy, hormones, immunotherapy, or biologics. In terms of malignant tumors, surgery plays a very limited role in tumor control. Mechanical instability has recently been defined for neoplastic disease and a Spine Instability Neoplastic Score (SINS) has been developed to aid in this assessment.[3] The recognition of spinal instability resulting from tumor is imperative because an unstable spine will not respond to radiation and/or chemotherapy but requires an intervention such as brace application, percutaneous cement augmentation and/or pedicle screws, or open surgery. The final assessment in NOMS reflects the extent of systemic disease, medical comorbidities, and expected survival, which all affect the decision to offer not only surgical treatment but also radiation or systemic therapy.

NOMS ASSESSMENT FOR NSCLC

The neurologic and oncologic assessments are considered together. From the oncologic perspective, radiation is the mainstay of therapy for tumor control because surgery and chemotherapy have little effect. It is unknown whether the newer biologics, such as erlotinib, have the same responses in bone metastases as visceral disease even if the epidermal growth factor receptor (EGFR) or other driver mutations are present. The two modalities of radiation currently available for the treatment of spine metastases are cEBRT and SRS. The neurologic assessment is one of the critical determinants in deciding between these modalities because cEBRT can be used in the setting of high-grade ESCC (ESCC 0–3) but the safe delivery of SRS requires a margin on the spinal cord to avoid radiation myelitis. Although investigators are studying the use of SRS in the setting of high-grade spinal cord compression, SRS use is usually restricted to tumors confined to the bone or with minimal epidural impingement (ESCC 0–1).[4,5]

NSCLC WITHOUT ESCC

A review of multiple series reporting histology-dependent responses demonstrate that NSCLC is generally resistant to cEBRT.[6–13] The response rates for radioresistant tumors, such as NSCLC, are reported between 20% to 33%, with the duration of the response reported at 1 to 3 months.[10,14] By contrast, NSCLC responds extremely well to SRS. A small number of series now report greater than 90% durable response rates when SRS is used as definitive treatment in patients with minimal or no spinal cord compression. In a review of 413 patients undergoing single-fraction SRS with doses ranging from 18 to 24 Gy, Yamada and colleagues[15] reported 3-year recurrence rates of 4% (when corrected for death). The NSCLC cohort had a 2% recurrence rate. Gerszten and colleagues[16] reviewed outcomes in 87 NCSLC patients treated with a maximum dose of 15 to 25 Gy delivered in a single fraction, and reported 89% pain improvement with no radiation toxicity. The application of SRS has transformed NSCLC into a relatively radiosensitive tumor.

NSCLC WITH HIGH-GRADE ESCC

From the neurologic and oncologic perspective, surgery is reserved for patients with NSCLC who have high-grade spinal cord compression. Surgery is used to preserve or restore neurologic function and stabilize the spine. The justification for surgery in patients with NSCLC is primarily based on a prospective randomized trial published by Patchell and colleagues[17] comparing surgery followed by cEBRT with cEBRT alone. The addition of surgery to cERBT was associated with statistically significant improvements in the maintenance and recovery of ambulation, bowel and bladder continence, narcotic requirements, and overall survival.

Although surgery provided neurologic salvage, durable tumor control remained a problem when using cEBRT as a postoperative adjuvant, with recurrence rates of approximately 70% at 1-year follow-up.[18] A major risk factor for recurrence is radioresistant-tumor histology. The transition to using SRS as a postoperative adjuvant has substantially improved local control rates compared with cEBRT, while reducing the need for aggressive surgical approaches. For metastatic disease, this new surgical approach is called separation surgery and is used to decompress the spinal cord and reconstitute the spinal fluid space in conjunction with a long screw-rod instrumented fusion.[19] Tumor in the vertebral body and large paraspinal masses are not resected, which reduces the time and morbidity from more extensive surgical approaches and aggressive tumor resection. This decompression provides a safe margin to deliver a cytotoxic radiation dose to the tumor within the constraints of spinal cord tolerance. In a review of 186 patients undergoing separation surgery with postoperative SRS, the 1-year estimated cumulative incidence of recurrence was 16.4%.[20] Patients receiving low-dose hypofractionated radiation (eg, 30 Gy in 5 fractions) had a local recurrence rate of 22.6%, compared with 4.1% and 9.0% after either high-dose hypofractionated (24–30 Gy in 3 fractions) or high-dose single fraction (24 Gy) SRS, respectively. Of the tumors treated, 144 (77%) were considered radioresistant to cEBRT and 91 (49%) had previously failed cEBRT. More aggressive approaches continue to be used selectively for both metastatic and superior sulcus tumors with spine involvement in which the entire vertebral body and/or chest wall are additionally resected. These techniques will be described in the surgical section.

MECHANICAL INSTABILITY

The assessment of mechanical instability is separate from the neurologic and oncologic assessments in the treatment of metastatic NSCLC to the spine. The recognition of instability creates a need for an interventional procedure, such as percutaneous cement augmentation of the vertebral body or open surgery. To aid clinicians in determining instability, the Spine Oncology Study Group recently reported the 18-point scoring system, SINS, based on systematic literature review and expert opinion.[3] In SINS, six parameters are considered to be the critical determinants in defining instability: location, pain, alignment, degree of osteolysis, presence of vertebral body collapse, and posterior element involvement. These parameters are weighted and the additive

point scores are used to determine if the spine is stable, potentially unstable, or unstable. Although SINS has been found to be both valid and reliable, the spine assessments required are very complicated for most surgeons who are not spine specialists, making it relatively impractical. However, from a clinical standpoint, the single best indicator of instability is the quality of the back or neck pain. Patients with spine tumors present with two predominant pain syndromes: biological or mechanical. Biological pain is nocturnal or early morning pain that resolves during the course of the day. It has been hypothesized to result from the diurnal variation in endogenous steroid secretion from the adrenal gland. Because of reduced steroid secretion at night, patients experience flare pain from inflammatory mediators secreted by the tumor. This pain is extremely responsive to exogenous steroid administration, and, ultimately, to definitive radiation treatment or surgical resection. By contrast, mechanical instability pain is typically present on movement or axial-load (ie, sitting or standing) and is level dependent. In the subaxial cervical spine (C3 to C7), instability is present on flexion and extension of the neck. In the atlantoaxial spine (occipital condyles to C2), patients additionally have rotational pain and often have severe occipital neuralgia (ie, pain radiating up the back of the head). However, patients with thoracic or thoracolumbar fractures often have pain when they lie flat because they extend an unstable kyphosis. These patients often prefer to sleep in a recliner, rather than to lie flat in bed. In the lumbar spine, instability is often associated with the syndrome of mechanical radiculopathy defined as axial load pain that causes severe back and leg pain. This syndrome is caused by collapse of the neural foramen on the exiting nerve root and requires surgical decompression of the facet joint and pedicle in addition to pedicle screw fixation.

Fortunately, most patients with mechanical instability resulting from NSCLC can be treated with percutaneous stabilization procedures. Percutaneous cement augmentation via techniques such as vertebroplasty or kyphoplasty significantly reduces pain in patients with pathologic compression fractures. Berenson and colleagues[21] reported the results of a multicenter prospective randomized trial comparing kyphoplasty to nonsurgical treatment of painful compression fractures. At 1 month after kyphoplasty there was significant improvement in the patients' functional status as assessed by the Roland-Morris Disability (RDQ) and SF-36 questionnaires, pain numeric rating score, and patient activity with reduction in bed rest days. The improvement was sustained at the 12-month follow-up, although the difference between the control and kyphoplasty groups lost statistical significance largely due to cross-over and slight improvement in the control group. No difference in complication rates was observed between the kyphoplasty and nonsurgical management groups. In the authors' experiences, patients with a pathologic compression fracture of the vertebral body with involvement of the posterior elements (facet joints or spinous processes) require posterior instrumentation in addition to vertebroplasty or kyphoplasty. Pedicle screws can now be placed percutaneously without the need for an extensive spine exposure (**Fig. 1**).

SYSTEMIC DISEASE AND MEDICAL COMORBIDITIES

The final assessment in the NOMS decision framework is the ability of the patient to tolerate a procedure based on the extent of systemic disease and medical comorbidities. After assessing the issues of neurologic, oncologic, and mechanical instability, the question remains whether the decision to intervene makes sense in the context of the patient's disease. Several factors are considered; however, the patient's life expectancy is foremost. Patients with spine metastases from NSCLC that require surgery for metastatic disease have reported median survival rates of only 4 months.[22] Short survivals can be predicted in many patients based on extensive visceral and bone disease, poor pulmonary function, and limited systemic options. However, many patients who have limited

systemic disease at the time of surgery die from rapid disease progression in the postoperative period. Epidural disease from NSCLC can be a harbinger of explosive systemic disease but in an unpredictable manner. This concept is critical to making decisions in this patient population, which is different from patients who present with metastatic disease early in their course or who have superior sulcus NSCLC that has responded well to induction chemoradiotherapy.

IMAGING SPINE TUMORS

Imaging for NSCLC is important in assessing the degree of bone, epidural, and paraspinal tumor. Thoracic surgeons typically use CT and CT–positron emission tomography (PET) for clinical staging of NSCLC. In the assessment of the spine, these are superb modalities for identifying the degree of bone destruction and as a screening tool to identify tumor. PET-CT can be used to differentiate tumor from benign bone lesions. In a review of patients who underwent 18-FDG-PET within 6 weeks of spine needle biopsy, the mean standardized uptake value (SUV) was 7.1 for malignant tumors compared with 2.1 for benign lesions ($P<.02$).[23] PET was a significantly better predictor of malignancy in nonsclerotic bone lesions. In lytic or mixed lytic-sclerotic bone lesions there was a 100% concordance between PET and needle biopsy with an SUV cutoff of 2.

Although CT and CT-PET are useful in assessing spine tumors, they do not address the issue of identifying and quantifying the degree of epidural tumor critical in decision making for NSCLC

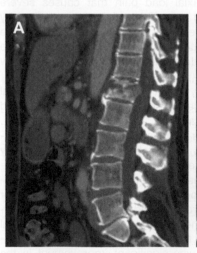 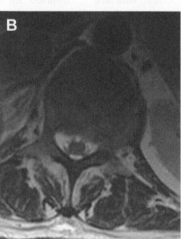 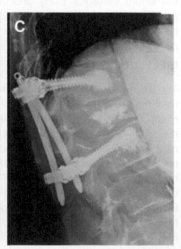

Fig. 1. Percutaneous screws. A 53-year-old woman with NSCLC presenting with severe back pain secondary to gross mechanical instability with SINS = 13. (*A*) Sagittal CT showing an osteolytic L1 metastasis. (*B*) Axial T2 and gadolinium-enhanced T1 MRI showing Grade Ib ESCC tumor with extension into the bilateral pedicles. (*C*) Patient underwent percutaneous T12-L2 screw fixation with cement augmentation and L1 kyphoplasty resulting in complete pain relief, followed by SRS to the L1 metastasis.

metastases and primary tumors with known or suspected vertebral body involvement. MRI is the most sensitive and specific modality for assessing spine tumors and should be ordered in cases in which tumor spine involvement is suspected. The extent of bone tumor and vertebral body involvement is best visualized using sagittal T1-weighted and STIR images. Typically, the entire spinal axis is imaged to assess for skip lesions or asymptomatic tumors that affect treatment. The degree of ESCC and paraspinal tumors are assessed using axial T2-weighted and T1-weighted postcontrast images.[2] The axial T2-weighted images produce a myelogram-effect that is very sensitive for assessing spinal cord compression, which is critical in decision making. More recently MRI perfusion images have been used to define the vascularity of tumors and responses to SRS specifically using plasma volume assessments.[24]

SURGICAL APPROACHES

As noted, the principal indication for open surgery with NSCLC involving the spine is high-grade ESCC. In the 1960s, laminectomy without instrumentation was used to treat spinal cord compression. At that time, multiple studies compared the results of noninstrumented laminectomy with cEBRT alone and failed to show superiority of the surgical treatment. Unfortunately, noninstrumented spinal decompression often exacerbated spinal instability in patients with vertebral tumor infiltration, thereby resulting in unfavorable surgical outcomes. Based on these data, cEBRT without surgery became the primary treatment of most patients with spinal metastases. With the development of spinal instrumentation, the results of spinal decompression in conjunction with instrumented stabilization in the treatment of spinal metastases were reassessed. Multiple surgical series demonstrated the safety and efficacy of instrumented spinal stabilization and decompression that can be accomplished using posterior, anterior, or combined approaches.[22,25] In the authors' practice, the midline posterior approach has become the workhorse for the treatment of metastatic spine disease. The posterior approach provides access to decompress and instrument the spine circumferentially. Epidural tumor and functional nerve roots can be dissected starting from normal dural planes. Additionally, transcavitary approaches are avoided with their inherent morbidity (eg, reduction of pulmonary function related to thoracotomy) as well as dissecting through previously operated or irradiated planes. Several posterior approaches have been described, including lateral extracavitary, costotransversectomy, and posterolateral laminectomy. Several ventral approaches continue to be used selectively in the metastatic population and for primary tumors involving the spine, such as superior sulcus tumors. In the thoracic spine, the anterior approach depends on the level of tumor involvement. Thoracotomy provides access to the ventral midthoracic and lower thoracic spine, whereas anterior transmanubrial or transsternal approaches may be required to access the upper thoracic spine. Access to the ventral spine allows complete or partial resection of the vertebral body and anterior spinal reconstruction using expandable or stackable cages or cement.[22,25]

SEPARATION SURGERY

The goals of spinal surgery in patients with metastatic tumors include decompression of the spinal cord and nerve root and spinal stabilization. Before popularization of spinal SRS, maximal tumor resection was undertaken to improve local control. Because spinal SRS has shown to provide reliable tumor control regardless of the tumor histology, volume, or prior radiation history, the goal of surgery has shifted from maximal cytoreduction to separation of the tumor from the dura and thus spinal cord, to allow safe postoperative SRS (**Fig. 2**). The separation of 2 to 3 mm between the tumor and the spinal cord is required to allow delivery of requisite radiation dose to the tumor without risking radiation toxicity to the spinal cord. This separation is provided by carrying out posterolateral laminectomies at the levels of epidural tumor extension and using the transpedicular approach to access the ventral epidural space. In this approach, a midline incision is made over the levels of intended decompression and instrumentation. The paraspinal muscles are dissected to expose the spinous processes, laminae, and transverse processes. Initially screw-rod constructs are placed a minimum of two levels superior and inferior to the level of the decompression. The decompression is accomplished with a 3-mm matchstick burr resecting the laminae, pedicles, and superior and inferior facet joints. Epidural tumor is resected beginning at normal dural planes beginning posterior. Tumor along the lateral dura is resected with tenotomy scissors, taking care to identify nerve roots exiting the common dural tube. Nerve roots are typically preserved but may be sacrificed by double ligating with vascular clips. Tumor extending into the ventral epidural space is resected in a piecemeal fashion and the posterior longitudinal ligament is sectioned to clear the dural margin of tumor.

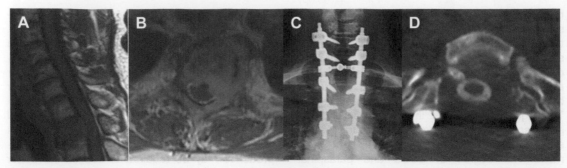

Fig. 2. Separation surgery. A 62-year-old man with NSCLC carcinoma presented with back pain and T2 metastasis with spinal cord displacement. (*A*) T1 sagittal and T1 gadolinium-enhanced MRI showing the T2 tumor with grade II ESCC. (*B*) Patient underwent separation surgery with T1-T3 laminectomy and C7-T5 posterolateral instrumentation and fusion. (*C*) Axial view of CT myelogram used for postoperative SRS planning showing circumferential decompression of the spinal cord and reconstitution of the CSF space around the spinal cord. (*D*) The 2-year follow-up MRI showing no evidence of tumor recurrence.

Resection of the vertebral body is usually not required to achieve a margin on the dura; however, the vertebral body can be resected through this posterior corridor using curettes and pituitary rongeur.

Spinal stabilization is carried out using posterior pedicle screws in the thoracic and lumbar spine or lateral mass screws in the subaxial spine. The instrumentation is usually placed at least two levels above and below the tumor. Tumor infiltrated levels are usually not instrumented due to significant risk of hardware pullout and fracture of the bone weakened by tumor. In patients with severe osteoporosis or diffuse osteolytic disease, screw purchase in bone may be reinforced using cement. The posterior construct has been shown to be a reliable stand-alone stabilization technique in patients with metastatic tumor. In patients with significant lysis of the vertebral body secondary to tumor invasion or extensive resection at the levels of decompression, anterior reconstruction may be carried out using combination of cement and Steinmann pins, cages, or allograft bone struts.

SUPERIOR SULCUS TUMORS WITH INVOLVEMENT OF THE SPINE

Superior sulcus tumors involving the spine are complicated by the extensive resection of supporting spine elements, the use of neoadjuvant chemoradiation, the need of cervicothoracic junction instrumentation, and the presence of comorbidities, including a prior history of smoking and osteoporosis. As opposed to metastatic disease, superior sulcus tumors invading the spine (T4) require both a posterior incision over the spine and a transthoracic approach (via a posterolateral thoracotomy). The incision must accommodate

bilateral exposure of the spine as well as a thoracotomy with elevation of the scapula. The authors' current practice is to make the vertical portion of the incision directly over the midline of the spine first and subsequently to "T" the thoracotomy incision for the more anterior approach. Moving the incision off the midline often puts the vertical incision over the ipsilateral hardware, increasing the risk of wound complications. The initial approach is via a posterolateral laminectomy with multilevel rhizotomy, and transverse process and proximal rib disarticulation from the spine. The C8 and T1 nerve roots are typically dissected from the neural foramen into the chest. Epidural tumor is resected from normal dural planes. The vertebral body can be resected from a posterior approach or delayed resection until the thoracotomy is performed. Posterior segmental fixation is placed, which requires instrumentation over the cervicothoracic junction, bridging the fixed thoracic to mobile cervical spine and transitioning from kyphosis to lordosis. The strategies for placing hardware include pedicle screw fixation with a 6.25 mm rod ending at C7 or a tapered rod construct bridging a 6.25 mm thoracic rod to a 3.5 mm cervical rod.[26] The wound is closed in layers. Following the posterior approach, the patient is turned from the prone to the lateral position and thoracotomy is performed with elevation of the scapula from the chest wall. The lateral rib osteotomies are created distal to the tumor and the upper lobectomy is completed. Critically, T1 is dissected from the T1-2 neural foramen to the junction of C8 and the lower trunk of the brachial plexus. In some cases, the T1 nerve root needs to be sacrificed, which may leave the patient with variable degrees of intrinsic hand weakness. Completion vertebrectomy is performed, followed by placement of an anterior strut using poly-methyl-methacrylate (PMMA) and

Steinman pins, titanium or polyether ether ketone (PEEK) cages, or auto or allograft struts. An anterior cervical plate or screw-rod construct can be placed to secure the anterior strut (**Fig. 3**).

Major Complications

Instrumentation failure
Improvements in spinal hardware provide excellent durable stabilization. Posterior hardware has evolved from sublaminar wires and hooks to screw-rod fixation. A recent review of 318 patients undergoing separation surgery with stand-alone posterior constructs revealed that only nine patients (2.8%) required revision of the hardware due to symptomatic hardware pull-out, rod break, or junctional fractures.[27] Two of the major risk factors for hardware failure were junctional tumors (ie, cervicothoracic tumor) and chest wall resection, both present in superior sulcus tumors. Several strategies are being implemented for these tumors, including cement augmentation of pedicle screws to provide better purchase and more aggressive reconstruction of the anterior column in at-risk patients.

Wound dehiscence or infection
One of the major risks of the posterior approach to the spine is wound infection or dehiscence. Major

risk factors in the cancer population include chemoradiation, instrumented fusion, and poor nutrition. In a series of 140 patients operated on for metastatic disease, the wound complication rate was 10.6%. Wound healing often occurred by secondary intention, which took months and delayed further therapy.[22] Attempts to shorten the healing time with vacuum-assisted closure frequently led to further complications with midline wound dehiscence over the hardware, especially at the cervicothoracic junction. The best solution has been the use of local muscle or myocutaneous flaps, including trapezius and latissimus turnover flaps for the cervical and thoracic spine, and local paraspinal advancement flaps for the lumbar spine. These often require only a single debridement, even in the setting of gross infection followed by a 6-week course of intravenous antibiotics. Covering metallic implants with nonirradiated vascularized tissue helps clear infection without the need to remove them. Vitaz and colleagues[28] reviewed 37 patients treated with rotational or transposition muscle or myocutaneous flaps. Patients underwent a mean of 1.3 procedures for the treatment of wound healing problems, despite positive cultures in 70%. In three patients (8%), this treatment failed due to protrusion of hardware through the skin or repeated dehiscence requiring reclosure.

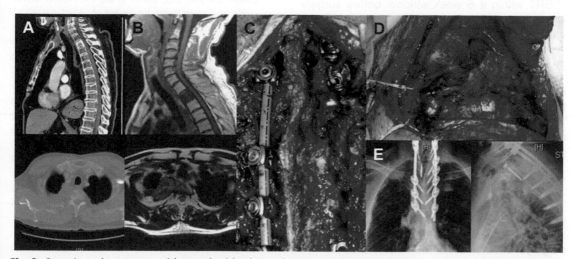

Fig. 3. Superior sulcus tumor with vertebral body involvement. A 54 year-old man with a 44 pack-year smoking history presents with 1-month history of right parascapular and arm pain extending to the wrist. Patient was diagnosed with a right superior sulcus mass extending into the T2 vertebral body. Needle biopsy was consistent with NSCLC. Clinical staging revealed a T4N0M0 tumor. Patient received induction chemoradiotherapy followed by a combined posterior approach and posterolateral thoracotomy. (*A*) CT: sagittal and axial images showing superior sulcus tumor with lytic destruction of T2 vertebral body. (*B*) MRI: T1-weighted sagittal and T2-weighted axial image demonstrating marrow infiltration but no ESCC. (*C*) Intraoperative picture showing at the posterior approach with left pedicle screw-rod placement and right T2 total facetectomy, T1 neurolysis, and T2 to 4 rhizotomy. (*D*) Intraoperative picture of the thoracotomy approach with the scapula elevated from the chest wall, T1 to 4 right rib resection, reconstructed vertebral body with methylmethacrylate and Steinman pins, and T1 extending to the lower trunk of the brachial plexus. (*E*) Plain radiograph AP and lateral showing the final pedicle screw and anterior reconstruction.

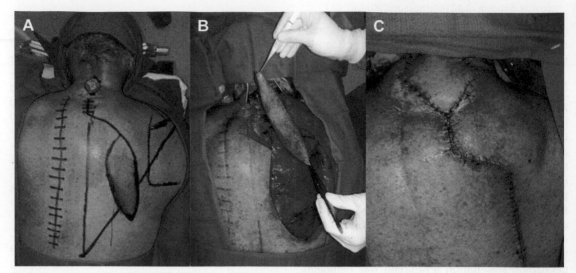

Fig. 4. A 70-year-old man with multiple recurrent tumors. The patient had a left trapezius myocutaneous flap at the time of initial tumor resection with adjuvant external beam radiation. Six years later he developed recurrent disease requiring re-resection. The postoperative course was complicated by lack of healing of the surgical site. A right trapezius myocutaneous flap was performed. (A) Preoperative image demonstrating nonhealing surgical site and markings showing the proposed left trapezius myocutaneous flap. Note the longitudinal scar on the right back (*hatched line*) following the previous trapezius flap. (B) Intraoperative image of the trapezius flap rotated. (C) Final intraoperative image.

Spinal instrumentation was salvaged in 97% of the cases. Patients who have been irradiated with cEBRT within a 6 week window before surgery are at highest risk for wound dehiscence. These patients should be considered for prophylactic flaps at the time of initial surgery (**Fig. 4**). The integration of SRS as a preoperative adjuvant should reduce the risk of wound dehiscence because the beams are targeted from multiple directions rather than directly through the wound as with cEBRT. This is reflected in a recent series in which the risk of infection or dehiscence was 17% in the cEBRT group versus 6% in the SRS group.[29]

SUMMARY

The NOMS considerations provide a dynamic decision framework to determine the optimal combination of systemic and radiation therapies and surgery. Generally, NSCLC metastases to the spine require SRS because cEBRT usually fails to provide consistent long-term local control. Patients with spinal cord compression secondary to NSCLC require surgical decompression to safely undergo SRS and to reduce the risk of radiation-induced spinal cord injury. Separation surgery allows spinal cord decompression and spinal stabilization using the posterior approach and, in combination with SRS, has been shown to provide reliable local control with low risk of wound complication or spinal hardware fracture.

REFERENCES

1. Laufer I, Rubin DG, Lis E, et al. The NOMS framework: approach to the treatment of spinal metastatic tumors. Oncologist 2013;18(6):744–51.
2. Bilsky MH, Laufer I, Fourney DR, et al. Reliability analysis of the epidural spinal cord compression scale. J Neurosurg Spine 2010;13(3):324–8.
3. Fisher CG, DiPaola CP, Ryken TC, et al. A novel classification system for spinal instability in neoplastic disease: an evidence-based approach and expert consensus from the Spine Oncology Study Group. Spine 2010;35(22):E1221–9.
4. Ryu S, Rock J, Jain R, et al. Radiosurgical decompression of metastatic epidural compression. Cancer 2010;116(9):2250–7.
5. Ryu S, Rock J, Rosenblum M, et al. Patterns of failure after single-dose radiosurgery for spinal metastasis. J Neurosurg 2004;101(Suppl 3):402–5.
6. Gerszten PC, Mendel E, Yamada Y. Radiotherapy and radiosurgery for metastatic spine disease: what are the options, indications, and outcomes? Spine 2009;34(Suppl 22):S78–92.
7. Gilbert RW, Kim JH, Posner JB. Epidural spinal cord compression from metastatic tumor: diagnosis and treatment. Ann Neurol 1978;3(1):40–51.
8. Maranzano E, Bellavita R, Rossi R, et al. Short-course versus split-course radiotherapy in metastatic spinal cord compression: results of a phase III, randomized, multicenter trial. J Clin Oncol 2005; 23(15):3358–65.

9. Maranzano E, Latini P. Effectiveness of radiation therapy without surgery in metastatic spinal cord compression: final results from a prospective trial. Int J Radiat Oncol Biol Phys 1995;32(4):959–67.

10. Maranzano E, Latini P, Perrucci E, et al. Short-course radiotherapy (8 Gy x 2) in metastatic spinal cord compression: an effective and feasible treatment. Int J Radiat Oncol Biol Phys 1997;38(5):1037–44.

11. Rades D, Fehlauer F, Schulte R, et al. Prognostic factors for local control and survival after radiotherapy of metastatic spinal cord compression. J Clin Oncol 2006;24(21):3388–93.

12. Rades D, Fehlauer F, Stalpers LJ, et al. A prospective evaluation of two radiotherapy schedules with 10 versus 20 fractions for the treatment of metastatic spinal cord compression: final results of a multicenter study. Cancer 2004;101(11):2687–92.

13. Rades D, Karstens JH, Alberti W. Role of radiotherapy in the treatment of motor dysfunction due to metastatic spinal cord compression: comparison of three different fractionation schedules. Int J Radiat Oncol Biol Phys 2002;54(4):1160–4.

14. Katagiri H, Takahashi M, Inagaki J, et al. Clinical results of nonsurgical treatment for spinal metastases. Int J Radiat Oncol Biol Phys 1998;42(5):1127–32.

15. Yamada Y, Cox B, Zelefsky MJ, et al. An analysis of prognostic factors for local control of malignant spine tumors treated with spine radiosurgery. Int J Radiat Oncol Biol Phys 2011;81(2S):S132–3.

16. Gerszten PC, Burton SA, Belani CP, et al. Radiosurgery for the treatment of spinal lung metastases. Cancer 2006;107(11):2653–61.

17. Patchell RA, Tibbs PA, Regine WF, et al. Direct decompressive surgical resection in the treatment of spinal cord compression caused by metastatic cancer: a randomised trial. Lancet 2005;366(9486):643–8.

18. Klekamp J, Samii H. Surgical results for spinal metastases. Acta Neurochir (Wien) 1998;140(9):957–67.

19. Moulding HD, Elder JB, Lis E, et al. Local disease control after decompressive surgery and adjuvant high-dose single-fraction radiosurgery for spine metastases. J Neurosurg Spine 2010;13(1):87–93.

20. Laufer I, Iorgulescu JB, Chapman T, et al. Local disease control for spinal metastases following "separation surgery" and adjuvant hypofractionated or high-dose single-fraction stereotactic radiosurgery:

21. outcome analysis in 186 patients. J Neurosurg Spine 2013;18(3):207–14.

21. Berenson J, Pflugmacher R, Jarzem P, et al. Balloon kyphoplasty versus non-surgical fracture management for treatment of painful vertebral body compression fractures in patients with cancer: a multicentre, randomised controlled trial. Lancet Oncol 2011;12(3):225–35.

22. Wang JC, Boland P, Mitra N, et al. Single-stage posterolateral transpedicular approach for resection of epidural metastatic spine tumors involving the vertebral body with circumferential reconstruction: results in 140 patients. Invited submission from the Joint Section Meeting on disorders of the spine and peripheral nerves, March 2004. J Neurosurg Spine 2004;1(3):287–98.

23. Laufer I, Lis E, Pisinski L, et al. The accuracy of [(18)F]fluorodeoxyglucose positron emission tomography as confirmed by biopsy in the diagnosis of spine metastases in a cancer population. Neurosurgery 2009;64(1):107–13.

24. Chu S, Karimi S, Peck KK, et al. Measurement of blood perfusion in spinal metastases with dynamic contrast-enhanced magnetic resonance imaging: evaluation of tumor response to radiation therapy. Spine 2013;38(22):E1418–24.

25. Walsh GL, Gokaslan ZL, McCutcheon IE, et al. Anterior approaches to the thoracic spine in patients with cancer: indications and results. Ann Thorac Surg 1997;64:1611–8.

26. Placantonakis DG, Laufer I, Wang JC, et al. Posterior stabilization strategies following resection of cervicothoracic junction tumors: review of 90 consecutive cases. J Neurosurg Spine 2008;9(2):111–9.

27. Amankulor NM, Xu R, Iorgulescu JB, et al. The incidence and patterns of hardware failure after separation surgery in patients with spinal metastatic tumors. Spine 2013;38(22):1623–9.

28. Vitaz TW, Oishi M, Welch WC, et al. Rotational and transpositional flaps for the treatment of spinal wound dehiscence and infections in patient populations with degenerative and oncological disease. J Neurosurg 2004;100(Suppl 1):45–51.

29. Keam J, Bilksy MH, Laufer I, et al. No association between excessive wound complications and preoperative high-dose hypofractionated, image-guided radiation therapy for spine metastasis. J Neurosug Spine 2014;20(4):411–20.

Pulmonary Resection After Pneumonectomy

Olaf Mercier, MD, Marc de Perrot, MD, Shaf Keshavjee, MD, FRCSC, FACS*

KEYWORDS

• Lung cancer • Recurrence • Pneumonectomy • Wedge resection • Surgery

KEY POINTS

- Limited lung resection for second primary lung cancer after pneumonectomy is a worthwhile procedure in appropriately selected patients that carries a low operative risk and allows for long-term survival, with a 5-year survival rate of up to 63%.
- Operations for metachronous cancers have a survival benefit that approximates the expected survival for primary lung cancer.
- The prognosis is poor for patients with N2 status and for those treated with a second surgery less than 2 years after the first procedure.
- Careful selection of potential candidates for remaining lung surgery is mandatory, with special attention given to cardiopulmonary reserve and lung cancer extension to achieve optimal early postoperative results and a long-term beneficial effect.
- Wedge resection with negative margins is the preferred procedure for peripheral tumors. Central tumors are best treated with segmentectomy.
- With the exception of middle lobectomy, lobectomy should be avoided because of its negative impact on cardiopulmonary reserve and outcomes.

INTRODUCTION

Second primary lung cancer is defined as a single lung lesion occurring after a prior resection. The risk of the development of second primary lung cancer in patients who survived after surgical resection of non–small cell lung cancer (NSCLC) is estimated to be 1% to 2% per patient per year.[1] This incidence has increased in recent years because of longer survival after resection of primary lung cancers and the widespread use of early detection tools, such as chest computed tomography (CT) and positron emission tomography (PET), during the postoperative follow-up. However, differentiating a second primary lung cancer from a metastatic lung cancer can be challenging, especially when a similar histology is found or if the recurrence is diagnosed relatively soon after the primary cancer. As the most referenced criteria for the definition of secondary primary lung cancers, Martini and Melamed's[2] indicators have been widely used by the medical community to help in such cases. Briefly, the criteria to diagnose a second primary lung cancer is indicated by a tumor-free interval of at least 2 years and a second cancer in a different lobe, lung, or origin from an area of carcinoma in situ, in the absence of other extrapulmonary or common lymphatic metastases.

The treatment of second primary lung cancer remains controversial because patients have

The authors have nothing to disclose.
Division of Thoracic Surgery, Toronto General Hospital, University Health Network, University of Toronto, 200 Elizabeth Street, 9N-946, Toronto, Ontario M5G 2C4, Canada
* Corresponding author.
E-mail address: shaf.keshavjee@uhn.ca

Thorac Surg Clin 24 (2014) 433–439
http://dx.doi.org/10.1016/j.thorsurg.2014.07.008
1547-4127/14/$ – see front matter © 2014 Elsevier Inc. All rights reserved.

already undergone surgery and new alternatives, such as stereotactic radiations and percutaneous ablations, have been available for the past few years. However, it has been demonstrated that surgical reresection could achieve satisfactory long-term survival with a low mortality rate in selected patients. Several investigators have reported a 5-year survival ranging from 23% to 60% after the resection of second primary lung cancers, with 0% to 5.8% postoperative mortality rate comparable with the first procedure.[3–6] One should emphasize that approximately two-thirds of patients experiencing second primary lung cancer could benefit from the surgery; the remaining one-third may not be eligible candidates for surgery because of advanced disease, comorbidities, or limited pulmonary reserve.[7]

Despite the evidence that reresection can achieve good oncologic outcomes with acceptable morbidity, surgical options have not been widely extended to patients who previously underwent pneumonectomy. Indeed, less than 100 cases have been reported in the literature to date, showing a 5-year survival of approximately 40% provided a limited resection was performed.[8–12] Specialists often do not consider subsequent additional lung resection after pneumonectomy for 2 reasons. First, pneumonectomy has a significant negative impact on pulmonary reserve and puts patients in a high-risk subgroup for lung resection. Second, surgical options are limited for stages higher than stage I given the fact that only sublobar resections can be safely performed.

The purpose of the authors' review is to report the early and long-term results of subsequent resection for lung cancer after pneumonectomy and to put it in perspective with the results of new increasing methods recently added to the field (stereotactic radiation and percutaneous ablation).

SELECTION OF PATIENTS FOR RESECTION

Defining good candidates for lung cancer resection after pneumonectomy remains a challenging clinical decision based on the evaluation of the benefit/risk ratio. The functional status of patients will impact the risk of the resection, whereas the lung cancer extension will impact the benefit of the procedure. Preoperative testing, such as pulmonary function tests and PET/CT, could help in evaluating the cardiopulmonary reserve and the tumoral extension.

Functional Status Evaluation and Cardiopulmonary Reserve

It is well established that patients who underwent a pneumonectomy have a limited cardiopulmonary reserve that could be similar to patients with chronic obstructive pulmonary disease with impaired lung function. Segmentectomy or extended wedge resection (with margins of 1 cm or equal to the tumor diameter) with hilar and mediastinal nodal evaluation is suggested by the American College of Chest Physicians and the Society of Thoracic Surgeons as a safe and effective alternative to lobectomy in high-risk patients with stage I NSCLC.[13] As a consequence, candidates for a second lung resection after pneumonectomy should have diagnosed clinical stage I NSCLC because a sublobar resection is the only feasible option. It has been described in the literature that additional lobectomy after pneumonectomy leads to increased postoperative mortality and worse long-term survival[14–16] with the exception of middle lobectomy after left pneumonectomy.[17] However, lobectomies after pneumonectomy were totally abandoned in the early 1990s; patients with stage I disease requiring a lobectomy because of its central position were deemed inoperable.

Even with limited resection, the negative impact of sublobar resection on pulmonary reserve in single-lung patients is comparable with the pulmonary impact achieved after lobectomy in patients with both lungs. Hence, careful evaluation of this reserve is required before making the decision to operate. The forced expiratory volume (FEV_1) and diffusing capacity of lung for carbon monoxide (DLCO) results accurately predict morbidity and mortality following major lung resection. Predicted postoperative (ppo) FEV_1 and ppoDLCO values less than 40% are useful to identify higher risk patients that may not benefit from the surgery. In this population, the assessment of peak oxygen consumption with exercise could be a better way to accurately evaluate the risk. In patients with ppoFEV$_1$ and/or ppoDLCO less than 40%, major resection was well tolerated if the peak oxygen consumption (p $\dot{V}_{o2}$) was greater than 10 mL/kg/min.[13]

The cardiac reserve assessment is also paramount. Because of the previous resection, the pulmonary vascular bed is reduced and additional lung resection may result in a dramatic increase in pulmonary artery pressure and right heart failure. Cardiac echography is a useful tool to screen any right heart dysfunction or pulmonary artery pressure elevation before the surgery. Right heart dysfunction and pulmonary hypertension are considered as absolute contraindications to resection.

In addition, health-related functional status and quality-of-life and comorbidity assessments are important for the treatment of single-lung patients with stage I NSCLC.

Non–Small Cell Lung Caner Extension Assessment

Confirmation of the malignant diagnosis and exclusion of metastatic disease are the most important issues to address. The use of PET has increased and proven to be a useful tool to suggest malignancy of a lung nodule, to screen for mediastinal lymph node involvement, and to diagnose distant metastases (**Fig. 1**). However, none of the 9 historical series on lung resection in single-lung patients reported the use of PET during the preoperative workup. Second primary lung cancer was defined using the Martini and Melamed[2] criteria based on the preoperative workup that included chest CT scan, bone scan, and brain CT scan as appropriate. The number of patients operated on for benign nodule over the same period of time (1984–2008) is not known. Grodzki and colleagues[12] were the only team to use a systematic percutaneous CT-guided biopsy with a positive result of 77% and no complications. It is prudent to try to avoid any useless surgery within this high-risk group of patients. Hence, diagnosis management of lung nodules in single-lung patients should not differ from that of patients with both lungs.

Preoperative mediastinal staging is necessary to substantially increase the benefit of the surgery. Indeed, better results are achieved in N0 compared with N2 lung cancers. Some investigators would suggest a systematic surgical mediastinal staging before the surgery considering the possible false-negative results of chest CT scan and PET.[6] However, in these cases, a mediastinoscopy could be challenging because of the aftereffects of previous surgeries and therapies: prior mediastinoscopy; mediastinal radiation therapy; pneumonectomy, which induces a mediastinal shift with tracheal displacement. For these reasons, endobronchial ultrasound seems to be the preferred method of mediastinal exploration.

In addition to chest CT scan, PET, and mediastinal staging, brain imaging is appropriate to rule out any brain metastases for patients at a higher risk for having metastatic disease. Brain magnetic resonance imaging or CT scan are appropriate for most of these patients.

Selecting patients with good pulmonary reserve and excluding patients with dissemination of the disease are the best guarantees for better long-term results and lower postoperative complication rates. Indications and contraindications of lung surgical resection after pneumonectomy are summarized in **Box 1**.

SURGICAL TECHNIQUE
Anesthetic Management

Postoperative pain control is paramount for good postoperative results and to facilitate a fast recovery while avoiding bronchial obstruction and atelectasis caused by ineffective cough, digestive complications caused by morphine overconsumption, and devastating postoperative pneumonia. Postoperative chest physiotherapy and early mobilization helps with bronchial clearance. An epidural catheter can be effective to reach

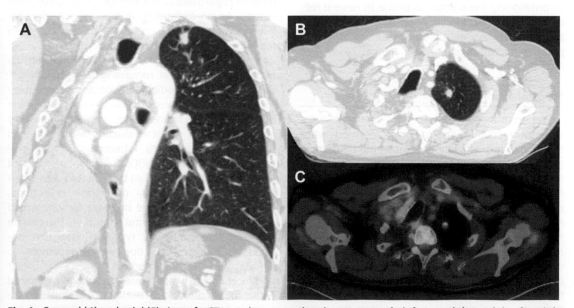

Fig. 1. Coronal (*A*) and axial (*B*) view of a CT scan demonstrating the presence of a left upper lobe nodule after right pneumonectomy. The PET scan (*C*) demonstrated uptake in the nodule suspicious for a new primary lung cancer.

Box 1
Indications and contraindications to lung resection after pneumonectomy

Indications

Diagnosis of second primary lung cancer

Clinical stage I disease

Sublobar resection feasible with good margins

Adequate cardiopulmonary reserve

Absolute contraindications

Greater than stage I disease

Lobectomy required (except middle lobectomy)

Pulmonary hypertension

Inadequate pulmonary reserve: ppoFEV$_1$ less than 40%, ppoDLCO less than 40%, p$\dot{V}_{o2}$ less than 10 mL/kg

Comorbidities limiting life expectancy to 2 years or less

Relative contraindications

Synchronous cancer

Metachronous cancer with disease-free interval of less than 2 years

Comorbidities increasing risk of surgery

these goals and reduce the amount of morphine given. Because patients have one lung remaining, the use of a double-lumen endotracheal tube is useless; a single-lumen endotracheal tube is usually inserted. Careful attention must be given to positioning the saturation probe to have a reliable signal during the entire procedure. An arterial line is useful for real-time assessment of intraoperative blood pressure and arterial blood gas assessment.

Surgical Procedure

Given that these patients have a single lung, surgical resection should be performed while the lung is still ventilating. Most of the time, minimizing the tidal volume using gentle hand ventilation and intermittent periods of apnea after hyperoxygenation allows for lung dissection, hilar dissection, sublobar resection, and mediastinal lymph node dissection. Some complex ventilation managements, including single lobe ventilation, high-frequency jet ventilation, and the use of extracorporeal membrane oxygenation,[10] have been described but are rarely useful because the aforementioned strategy is reliable and effective with close collaboration between the anesthesiologist and the surgeon.

The preferred approaches for patients undergoing pulmonary resection after pneumonectomy are either median sternotomy or thoracotomy. The inability to sustain apnea more than a few minutes precludes the possibility of using video-assisted thoracic surgery. However, limited muscle-sparing thoracotomy could be used as a minimally invasive approach for small peripheral nodules that could be resected with good margins with wedge resection. Standard thoracotomy sparing the anterior serratus is the most popular approach allowing for lung palpation, segmentectomy, and lymph node dissection with a good level of safety. This approach is particularly used for central tumors requiring segmentectomy and posterior tumors. Anterior tumors from the upper and middle lobes could be approached through a median sternotomy given the mediastinal shift induced by the previous pneumonectomy. It gives the advantage of limiting the post-thoracotomy pain but makes the lymph node dissection more challenging.

The extent of pulmonary resection is determined by the size, depth, and location of the lung cancer to be resected. Lung-sparing oncological surgery principles are the general rules of modern thoracic surgery. However, when resection after pneumonectomy is needed, the lung conservation should be more important than usual, keeping in mind that complete resection is mandatory. Resections more extensive than a sublobar resection have been associated with a worse survival rate.[8,14–16] Poor outcomes of lobectomy after pneumonectomy represent a limitation of pulmonary vascular reserve regardless of the preoperative spirometric values. As an exception, middle lobectomy after left pneumonectomy could be considered safe for a central middle lobe lesion, essentially accomplishing a bisegmentectomy with a relatively small impact on the remaining lung function.[17] Evidence-based medicine advocates segmentectomy or extended wedge resection (with margins of 1 cm or equal to the tumor diameter) with hilar and mediastinal nodal evaluation as a safe and effective alternative to lobectomy in high-risk patients with stage I NSCLC.[13] Hence, most of the peripheral lesions could be resected with satisfactory margins by way of wedge resections. Conversely, more central or large tumors would require anatomic segmental resection. The choice between these different types of resection depends on the surgeon's operative assessment.

As stated by the American consensus,[13] hilar and mediastinal lymph nodes should be evaluated either by complete dissection or sampling according to the thoracic surgeon in charge of the patients.

Table 1
International experience reports published between 1985 and 2013 on surgical management of second lung cancer after prior pneumonectomy

Author Name, Ref. Year	No. Patients	Time to Recurrence	Preop FEV$_1$ (%)	Resections	Mortality (%)	Overall 5-y Survival (%)	Metachronous Survival (%)
Kittle et al,[14] 1985	15	57 (4–192)	NA	9 Wedges / 5 Segments / 1 Lobectomy	8	18	NA
Levasseur et al,[15] 1992	9	56 (2–170)	NA	5 Wedges / 1 Segment / 3 Lobectomies	33	14 (2-y)	NA
Westermann et al,[16] 1993	8	45 (14–135)	NA	2 Wedges / 5 Segments / 1 Lobectomy	16	20 (3-y)	NA
Massard et al,[17] 1995	4	36 (12–71)	62 (52–80)	1 Wedge / 1 Segment / 2 Lobectomies	0	25	NA
Spaggiari et al,[11] 1996	13	38 (9–90)	NA	9 Wedges / 3 Segments / 1 Exploration	0	46 (3-y)	NA
Terzi et al,[9] 1997	7	28	NA	6 Wedges / 1 Segment	0	15	NA
Donington et al,[8] 2002	24	23 (2–213)	43 (29–83) (ppo)	20 Wedges / 3 Segments / 1 Lobectomy	8.3	40	50
Terzi,[10] 2004	14	35 (11–264)	59 (46–80)	12 Wedges / 2 Segments	0	37	45
Grodzki et al,[12] 2008	18	18 (4–106)	63 ± 14	18 Wedges	—	44	63

Abbreviations: NA, not available; Preop, preoperative.
Data from Refs.[8–12,14–17]

CLINICAL OUTCOMES

Over the past 30 years, 8 peer-reviewed reports and one correspondence were published on outcomes of lung resection after a previous pneumonectomy[8–12,14–17] including a total of 112 patients (Table 1). Most of the resections were sublobar resections: 74% wedge resection, 18% segmentectomy, and 8% lobectomy (5 of 7 were middle lobectomies); the long-term survival outcomes confirmed that in these high-risk patients, limited resection provides the best risk-benefit ratio. The postoperative mortality decreased from 13.8% (for the first 4 series) to (2.6% for the last 5 series). Of interest, most of the mortality in the early experience was caused by respiratory failure related to the extent of lung resection greater than a segmentectomy or a wedge. The mean interval time between the pneumonectomy and the resection of the second primary lung cancer ranged from 2 months to more than 15 years. The first series included in their survival results early recurrence (before 2 years, eg, stage IV NSCLC) and late recurrence (metachronous disease, eg, real second primary NSCLC), partially explaining their worse survival. The last 3 series separated the survival of metachronous disease, which demonstrated a 5-year survival rate ranging from 45% to 63%.[8–10,12] Considering only these last series, which included half of the patients (56 patients) who complied with the most recent guidelines for lung cancer care, the overall 5-year survival rates ranged from 37% to 44%. Two predictors of poor prognosis have been found: N2 status and the time interval between surgeries (early vs metachronous).[12]

ALTERNATIVES TO SURGICAL MANAGEMENT

Because surgical resection after pneumonectomy is worthwhile for highly selected patients, other techniques have emerged during the last decade for patients deemed inoperable. The first technique is stereotactic body radiotherapy (SBRT), which refers to the highly precise and accurate delivery of very conformal and dose-intensive radiation to small-volume targets. The recent Radiation Therapy Oncology Group trial (RTOG 0236)[18] enrolled a homogeneous population with biopsy-proven inoperable stage I NSCLC treated with 60 Gy in 3 fractions. Indicators defining inoperability included FEV_1 less than 40%; $ppoFEV_1$ less than 30%; DLCO less than 40%; hypoxemia or hypercapnia; pulmonary hypertension; diabetes with end-organ damage or severe cerebral, cardiovascular, or peripheral vascular disease; or chronic heart disease. An overall survival of 56% at 3 years was achieved. The first report using SBRT for the treatment of second primary NSCLC after pneumonectomy was published in 2009.[19] The investigators reported the outcomes of 15 patients presenting with an inoperable second primary lung cancer after prior pneumonectomy. The maximum tumor diameters ranged between 8 and 38 mm, and no local failures were diagnosed after a median follow-up of 16.5 months. The results of this series were updated in 2013,[20] showing a median survival of 39 months, a recurrence rate of 15%, and a 3-year survival of 63%. SBRT seems to be a promising alternative in inoperable patients with stage I NSCLC after pneumonectomy. However, patients' follow-ups are still limited in time; and long-term survival (5-year survival) may not remain as high as the 3-year survival. In addition, even if SBRT is convenient for peripheral stage I tumors, central tumors and tumors of more than 3 cm remained a matter of concern because radiation is limited because of the lung toxicity contraindicating SBRT. Taking these results together, SBRT seems to be a promising technique for inoperable postpneumonectomy patients with peripheral second stage I NSCLC.

Percutaneous ablative therapy (radiofrequency, cryoablation) seems to be a less promising alternative technique considering the high rate of pneumothorax, pleural effusion, and hemoptysis following this procedure (15%–55%) and the reduced primary tumor control (relapse rate 8%–43%).[13] However, Yamauchi[21] reported 2 cases of percutaneous cryoablation of secondary small peripheral NSCLC in postpneumonectomy patients that achieved local control for 2 and 4 years, respectively, without any complication at the time of the procedure and without damage to the remaining lung.

SUMMARY

Limited lung resection for second primary lung cancer after pneumonectomy is a worthwhile procedure in appropriately selected patients because it carries a low operative risk and allows for long-term survival with good quality of life. Operations for metachronous cancers had a survival benefit that approximated the expected survival for primary lung cancer. The prognosis is poor for patients with N2 status and for those treated by second surgery earlier than 2 years after the first procedure. Careful selection of potential candidates for remaining lung surgery with special attention to functional cardiopulmonary reserve and lung cancer extension is mandatory for optimal early postoperative results and a long-term beneficial effect. Wedge resection with negative margins is the preferred procedure for peripheral tumors. Central tumors would benefit more from segmentectomy. With the exception of middle lobectomy, lobectomy should be avoided because of its negative impact on cardiopulmonary reserve and outcomes. In highly selected patients, surgical resection of a second primary NSCLC after pneumonectomy following these principles may achieve a 5-year survival rate of up to 63%. SBRT has shown promising early results as an alternative to surgical resection in inoperable patients.

REFERENCES

1. Johnson BE. Second lung cancers in patients after treatment for an initial lung cancer. J Natl Cancer Inst 1998;90(18):1335–45.
2. Martini N, Melamed MR. Multiple primary lung cancers. J Thorac Cardiovasc Surg 1975;70(4):606–12.
3. Battafarano RJ, Force SD, Meyers BF, et al. Benefits of resection for metachronous lung cancer. J Thorac Cardiovasc Surg 2004;127(3):836–42.
4. Bae MK, Byun CS, Lee CY, et al. The role of surgical treatment in second primary lung cancer. Ann Thorac Surg 2011;92(1):256–62.
5. Hamaji M, Allen MS, Cassivi SD, et al. Surgical treatment of metachronous second primary lung cancer after complete resection of non–small cell lung cancer. J Thorac Cardiovasc Surg 2013;145(3):683–91.
6. Wood DE. Pulmonary resection after pneumonectomy. Thorac Surg Clin 2004;14(2):173–82.
7. Rice DC, Erasmus JJ, Stevens CW, et al. Extended surgical staging for potentially resectable malignant pleural mesothelioma. Ann Thorac Surg 2005;80(6):1988–93.
8. Donington JS, Miller DL, Rowland CC, et al. Subsequent pulmonary resection for bronchogenic carcinoma after pneumonectomy. Ann Thorac Surg 2002;74(1):154–8 [discussion: 158–9].
9. Terzi A, Furlan G, Gorla A, et al. Lung resection on single residual lung after pneumonectomy for bronchogenic carcinoma. Thorac Cardiovasc Surg 1997;45(6):273–6.
10. Terzi A. Lung resection for bronchogenic carcinoma after pneumonectomy: a safe and worthwhile procedure. Eur J Cardiothorac Surg 2004;25(3):456–9.
11. Spaggiari L, Grunenwald D, Girard P, et al. Cancer resection on the residual lung after pneumonectomy for bronchogenic carcinoma. Ann Thorac Surg 1996;62(6):1598–602.
12. Grodzki T, Alchimowicz J, Kozak A, et al. Additional pulmonary resections after pneumonectomy: actual long-term survival and functional results. Eur J Cardiothorac Surg 2008;34(3):493–8.
13. Donington J. American College of Chest Physicians and Society of Thoracic Surgeons consensus statement for evaluation and management for high-risk patients with stage I non-small cell lung cancer. Chest 2012;142(6):1620.
14. Kittle CF, Faber LP, Jensik RJ, et al. Pulmonary resection in patients after pneumonectomy. Ann Thorac Surg 1985;40(3):294–9.
15. Levasseur P, Regnard JF, Icard P, et al. Cancer surgery on a single residual lung. Eur J Cardiothorac Surg 1992;6(12):639–40 [discussion: 641].
16. Westermann CJ, van Swieten HA, Brutel de la Rivière A, et al. Pulmonary resection after pneumonectomy in patients with bronchogenic carcinoma. J Thorac Cardiovasc Surg 1993;106(5):868–74.
17. Massard G, Wihlm JM, Morand G. Surgical management for metachronous bronchogenic cancer occurring after pneumonectomy. J Thorac Cardiovasc Surg 1995;109(3):597–600.
18. Timmerman R, Paulus R, Galvin J, et al. Stereotactic body radiation therapy for inoperable early stage lung cancer. JAMA 2010;303(11):1070–6.
19. Haasbeek CJ, Lagerwaard FJ, de Jaeger K, et al. Outcomes of stereotactic radiotherapy for a new clinical stage I lung cancer arising postpneumonectomy. Cancer 2009;115(3):587–94.
20. Senthi S, Haasbeek CJ, Lagerwaard FJ, et al. Radiotherapy for a second primary lung cancer arising post-pneumonectomy: planning considerations and clinical outcomes. J Thorac Dis 2013;5(2):116–22.
21. Yamauchi Y. Percutaneous cryoablation for pulmonary nodules in the residual lung after pneumonectomy. Chest 2011;140(6):1633.

beneficial effect. Wedge resection with negative margins is the preferred procedure for peripheral tumors. Central tumors would benefit more from segmentectomy. With the exception of middle lobectomy, lobectomy should be avoided because of its negative impact on cardiopulmonary reserve and outcomes. In highly selected patients, surgical resection of a second primary NSCLC after pneumonectomy following these principles may achieve a 5-year survival rate of up to 63%. SBRT has shown promising early results as an alternative to surgical resection in inoperable patients.

REFERENCES

Superior Vena Caval Resection in Lung Cancer

Dong-Seok D. Lee, MD*, Raja M. Flores, MD

KEYWORDS

- Lung cancer • Superior vena cava • Caval invasion • Caval resection • Caval reconstruction

KEY POINTS

- Superior vena caval (SVC) invasion has been downstaged to reflect potential resectability with the most recent staging classification.
- Patterns of involvement include central tumor or metastatic mediastinal lymph nodes.
- En bloc resection may require tangential or complete SVC resection.
- Reconstruction may entail simple suture repair or a prosthesis.
- Five-year survival rates can reach up to 30%.

INTRODUCTION

Lung cancer is the leading cause of cancer death worldwide. Surgical resection remains the mainstay of treatment of early-stage disease. Involvement of the superior vena cava (SVC) in lung carcinoma has traditionally been considered a contraindication for surgical resection. These patients have historically been classified as stage IIIB disease, with a 5-year survival of up to 8%.[1]

BACKGROUND

Over the past 30 years, reports in the literature have challenged this notion. Patients undergoing SVC resection with reconstruction in the setting of lung cancer have reported 5-year survival rates up to 30% (**Table 1**). Therefore, the most recent iteration of the staging system has taken this into account and has transferred T4N0–1M0 tumors into stage IIIA disease.

Superior vena cava involvement encompasses a spectrum of diseases. The SVC can be involved through either direct invasion of central tumors (T4 disease) or invasion of metastatic lymph nodes (N2 disease). In addition, it can be involved in isolation or in conjunction with other mediastinal structures. Patients may present with SVC syndrome.

PREOPERATIVE EVALUATION

Comprehensive preoperative evaluation is imperative in determining whether a patient is an appropriate surgical candidate. A concerted effort should be made to determine whether N2 disease is present through diagnostic imaging and possibly diagnostic biopsies. Sites of distant disease preclude surgical resection. Preoperative pulmonary function testing is essential, because resection may necessitate pneumonectomy. In addition, the phrenic nerve is often sacrificed with complete SVC resection; thus, bilateral phrenic nerve involvement is a contraindication to resection.

THERAPEUTIC OPTIONS AND/OR SURGICAL TECHNIQUES

The surgical approach is based on surgeon preference. Most resections can be performed via a standard posterolateral thoracotomy, but other

Disclosure: Neither author has any conflicts of interest to disclose.
Department of Thoracic Surgery, Mount Sinai Health System, Icahn School of Medicine at Mount Sinai, One Gustave L. Levy Place, Box 1023, New York, NY 10029, USA
* Corresponding author.
E-mail address: dong-seok.lee@mountsinai.org

Thorac Surg Clin 24 (2014) 441–447
http://dx.doi.org/10.1016/j.thorsurg.2014.07.009
1547-4127/14/$ – see front matter Published by Elsevier Inc.

Table 1
Results of SVC resection and reconstruction in the setting of lung cancer from selected case series

Author	Patients	Morbidity (%)	Mortality (%)	Median Survival	5-Year Survival (%)
Lanuti et al,[8] 2009	9			21.4 mo	31.0
Suzuki et al,[7] 2004	40	40.0	10.0		24.0
Shargall et al,[6] 2004	15		14.0	40.0 mo	57.0 (3-y)
Sekine et al,[9] 2010	9				18.8
Thomas et al,[10] 1994	15	20.0	7.0	8.5 mo	24.0
Yildizeli et al,[5] 2008	39	10.3	7.7	19.0 mo	29.4
Misthos et al,[11] 2007	9		0	31.0 mo	11.0
Spaggiari et al,[12] 2004	109	30.0	12.0	11.0 mo	21.0

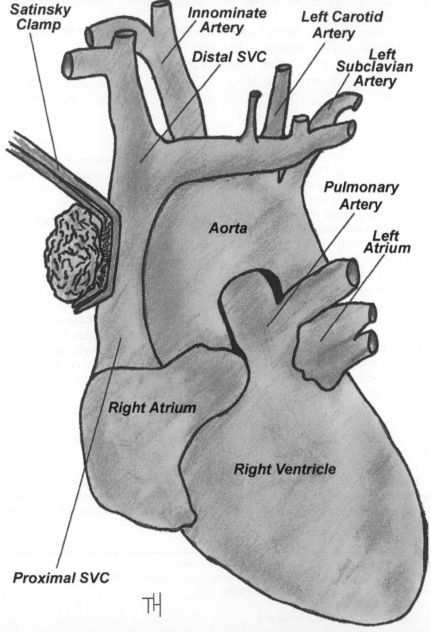

Fig. 1. A partial occlusion clamp is placed over a small tumor invading the SVC for vascular control. (*From* Garcia A, Flores RM. Surgical management of tumors invading the superior vena cava. Ann Thorac Surg 2008;85:2144; with permission.)

approaches include median sternotomy, hemiclam-shell thoracotomy, cervicosternotomy, and combined cervicotomy and thoracotomy. Large-bore intravenous access in the lower extremity is necessary to maintain volume during SVC clamping.

Superior vena caval resection and reconstruction can be performed through tangential or complete resection. When only a small portion of the SVC is involved, a partial occlusion clamp can be used for vascular control with subsequent en bloc resection. Depending on the size of the defect, a primary suture repair can be attempted or patch repair can be performed with autologous pericardium or prosthesis (**Figs. 1** and **2**). This

technique avoids the risk of potential future graft infection. If more than 50% of the diameter of the SVC requires resection, a graft replacement becomes necessary.

In the case of complete resection, total SVC clamping is necessary for vascular control. Attempts should be made to clamp the SVC above the azygos vein to preserve some flow to limit brain anoxia. However, if tumor anatomy makes this impossible, the SVC can be clamped for up to 60 minutes based on experimental animal models.[2]

Patients with extensive collateralization of flow from chronic SVC syndrome have few hemodynamic sequelae from cross-clamping. However,

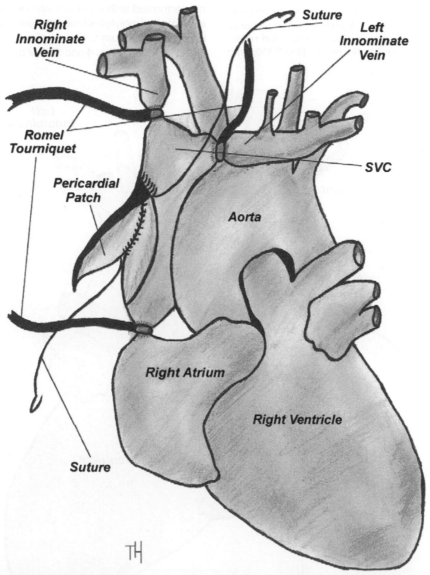

Fig. 2. Patch repair of SVC wall with autologous pericardium. (*From* Garcia A, Flores RM. Surgical management of tumors invading the superior vena cava. Ann Thorac Surg 2008;85:2144; with permission.)

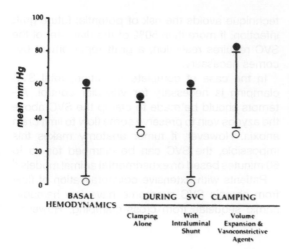

Fig. 3. Hemodynamic changes during cross-clamping of the SVC. (*From* Dartevelle P, Macchiarini P, Chapelier A. Technique of superior vena cava resection and reconstruction. Chest Surg Clin North Am 1995;5:350; with permission.)

acute occlusion of the patent SVC with a clamp can induce several adverse hemodynamic effects. Decreased right ventricular preload results in decreased cardiac output and eventual systemic hypotension. In addition, increased venous pressure can increase the risk of intracranial thrombosis and edema. This combination can result in irreversible brain damage. Therefore, given these potential hemodynamic effects, patients presenting with acute SVC obstruction should never be considered for urgent SVC resection. These hemodynamic effects are usually self-limiting and can be minimized intraoperatively with intravascular fluid expansion and vasoconstrictive agents (**Fig. 3**).[3]

Complete SVC resection and reconstruction can be performed with an in situ interposition graft using a ringed polytetrafluoroethylene graft or tubularized pericardium with or without a caval shunt after resection (**Figs. 4** and **5**). For tumors involving

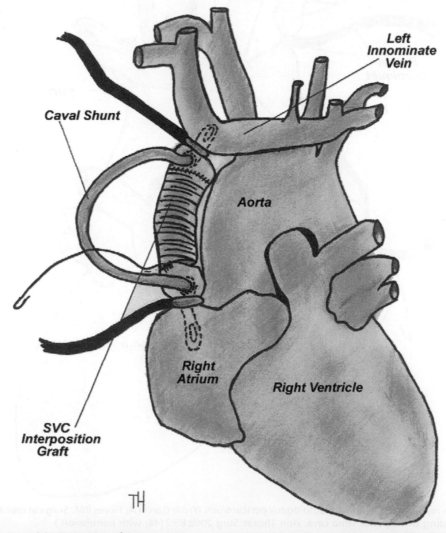

Fig. 4. Resection of the SVC with graft interposition using a ringed polytetrafluoroethylene graft. (*From* Garcia A, Flores RM. Surgical management of tumors invading the superior vena cava. Ann Thorac Surg 2008;85:2145; with permission.)

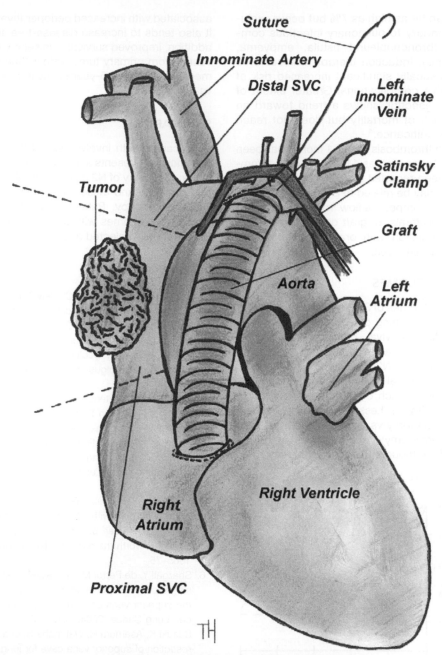

Fig. 5. A graft is sewn from the right atrium to the left innominate vein before tumor resection. SVC, superior vena cava. (*From* Garcia A, Flores RM. Surgical management of tumors invading the superior vena cava. Ann Thorac Surg 2008;85:2145; with permission.)

the proximal SVC and the right innominate vein, the graft may be placed between the left innominate vein and the right atrium, followed by SVC resection. Only one innominate venous drainage needs to be preserved, because the unilateral arm swelling seen with transection of one vein resolves over time. Systemic heparinization is sometimes recommended, but the authors do not routinely heparinize. Cardiopulmonary bypass is usually not necessary.

COMPLICATIONS AND CONCERNS

Postoperative morbidity and mortality can be as high as 40% and 14%, respectively. Most complications are respiratory. Incidence of graft infection can be as high as 7% but occur exclusively secondary to pulmonary infectious complications (bronchopleural fistula, empyema, lung abscess). Induction therapy is associated with a statistically significant increased risk of postoperative complications. Greater extent of pulmonary resection shows a trend toward an increased risk of mortality but does not reach statistical significance.[4]

Early graft thrombosis (within 1 month) has been reported to be as high as 11%. Late graft thrombosis has been reported as high as 30%. Risk of thrombosis may be related to SVC stenosis in primary repairs, competitive flow from extra grafts or extensive collaterals, or graft caliber. Postoperative anticoagulation with oral warfarin for 3 to 6 months is often given.

CLINICAL OUTCOMES

Long-term outcomes of SVC resection and reconstruction in the setting of advanced lung cancer yields median survival ranging from 8.5 to 40.0 months, with a 5-year survival rate up to 30%. Patients with N2 disease show a trend toward worse survival outcomes than those with N0/N1 disease, which does not reach statistical significance (**Fig. 6**). Lesser extent of pulmonary resection (lobectomy vs pneumonectomy vs carinal pneumonectomy) also improves long-term outcomes.[5] Although induction therapy was

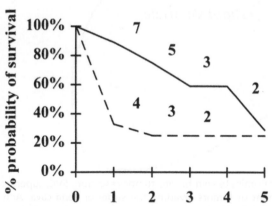

Fig. 6. Survival curves (actuarial method) of patients with N0–1 lymph node involvement (*continuous curve*) or N2 involvement (*dotted curve*) and SVC system resection for T4, non-small cell lung cancer. The numbers along the curves indicate the patients alive and still at risk at the corresponding date. The 5-year probabilities of survival were 30% and 25%, respectively. The comparison by log-rank test was not significant. (*From* Spaggiari L, Regnard JF, Magdeleinat P, et al. Extended resections for bronchogenic carcinoma invading the superior vena cava system. Ann Thorac Surg 2000;69:235; with permission.)

associated with increased perioperative morbidity, it also tends to increase disease-free survival.[6] In addition, improved survival was seen with SVC invasion from primary tumor rather than metastatic mediastinal nodes (5-year survival rates of 36.0% vs 6.6%).[7]

SUMMARY

Lung cancer with involvement of the SVC is uncommon but presents a unique management challenge. Discovery of N2 disease should be given its due diligence and these patients should undergo induction therapy. Patients can attain favorable long-term outcomes with surgery, but they need to be carefully selected at specialized centers.

REFERENCES

1. Tanoue LT, Detterbeck FC. New TNM classification for non-small-cell lung cancer. Expert Rev Anticancer Ther 2009;9:413–23.
2. Masuda H, Ogata T, Kikuchi K. Physiologic changes during temporary occlusion of the superior vena cava in cynomolgus monkeys. Ann Thorac Surg 1989;47:890–6.
3. Dartevelle PG. Extended operations for the treatment of lung cancer. Ann Thorac Surg 1997;63:12–9.
4. Spaggiari L, Thomas P, Magdeleinat P, et al. Superior vena cava resection with prosthetic replacement for non-small cell lung cancer: long term results of a multicentric study. Eur J Cardiothorac Surg 2002;21: 1080–6.
5. Yildizeli B, Dartevelle PG, Fadel E, et al. Results of primary surgery with T4 non-small cell lung cancer during a 25-year period in a single center: the benefit is worth the risk. Ann Thorac Surg 2008;86: 1065–75.
6. Shargall Y, de Perrot M, Keshavjee S, et al. 15 years single center experience with surgical resection of the superior vena cava for non-small cell lung cancer. Lung Cancer 2004;45:357–63.
7. Suzuki K, Asamura H, Watanabe S, et al. Combined resection of superior vena cava for lung carcinoma: prognostic significance of patterns of superior vena cava invasion. Ann Thorac Surg 2004;78:1184–9.
8. Lanuti M, De Delva PE, Gaissert HA, et al. Review of superior vena cava resection in the management of benign disease and pulmonary or mediastinal malignancies. Ann Thorac Surg 2009;88:392–8.
9. Sekine Y, Suzuki H, Saitoh Y, et al. Prosthetic reconstruction of the superior vena cava for malignant disease: surgical techniques and outcomes. Ann Thorac Surg 2010;90:223–8.
10. Thomas P, Magnan PE, Moulin G, et al. Extended operation for lung cancer invading the superior vena cava. Eur J Cardiothorac Surg 1994;8:177–82.

11. Misthos P, Papagiannakis G, Kokotsakis J, et al. Surgical management of lung cancer invading the aorta or the superior vena cava. Lung Cancer 2007;56: 223–7.

12. Spaggiari L, Magdeleinat P, Kondo H, et al. Results of superior vena cava resection for lung cancer: analysis of prognostic factors. Lung Cancer 2004; 44:339–46.

Surgical Resection of Non–Small Cell Lung Cancer with N2 Disease

Jessica S. Donington, MD*, Harvey I. Pass, MD

KEYWORDS

- Non–small cell lung cancer • Resection • Stage IIIA • Mediastinal lymph nodes

KEY POINTS

- Stage IIIa non–small cell lung cancer with mediastinal lymph node involvement comprises a large and heterogeneous population; the role of surgery in treatment algorithms is determined by the bulk and extent of mediastinal lymph node disease.
- In patients with clinical N2, surgery alone is not appropriate and induction therapy is the standard of care.
- Clearance of disease from the mediastinal lymph nodes by induction therapy is an important marker for improved survival after resection.
- The choice of induction regimens is widely debated. Although concurrent chemotherapy and radiation appears to be associated with increased mediastinal nodal clearance, it also appears to be associated with increased operative morbidity and mortality when used in combination with resections more extensive than a lobectomy, and, therefore, needs to be used selectively.

INTRODUCTION

Almost one-third of all patients diagnosed with non–small cell lung cancer (NSCLC) present with locally advanced disease. Most of these patients are treated for cure, but there are many treatment options and they can vary considerably. All curative treatment plans are multimodality in nature, because of the need to address both the localized disease and the high risk for occult metastatic disease. Systemic chemotherapy is used to address the incredibly large risk for distal spread and represents the backbone of treatment strategies, but there is currently little consensus on the optimal modality for local therapy. Both surgery and radiation have important roles, but protocols for their integration with chemotherapy remains greatly debated. T1–3 tumors with N2 involvement represent the largest cohort of patients with stage IIIA and are the group in whom the most controversy exists as to the role of surgery. Over the past 3 decades, our understanding of which patients with N2 disease benefit from resection and which patients surgery provides increased toxicity without survival benefit has grown tremendously. This text focuses on approach and outcomes for surgical resection in patients with stage IIIA disease who have N2 (ipsilateral medistinall) lymph node involvement.

EXTENT OF N2 DISEASE

Despite several decades of clinical trials attempting to address the topic, the role of surgery for patients with N2 disease remains provocative. Most would agree that any benefit of surgery is limited

The authors have nothing to disclose.
Department of Cardiothoracic Surgery, NYU School of Medicine, 530 1st Avenue, Suite 9V, New York, NY 10016, USA
* Corresponding author.
E-mail address: jessica.donington@nyumc.org

Thorac Surg Clin 24 (2014) 449–456
http://dx.doi.org/10.1016/j.thorsurg.2014.07.010
1547-4127/14/$ – see front matter © 2014 Elsevier Inc. All rights reserved.

to those who undergo a complete resection and all involved mediastinal disease can be removed. Incomplete resections and tumor debulking do not provide a survival benefit. From a surgical standpoint, N2 involvement can be divided into 3 broad categories: (1) incidental or occult, (2) discrete or potentially resectable, and (3) bulky unresectable or infiltrative disease. Incidental or occult N2 involvement describes that found at the time of surgery in patients who were clinical N0 or N1 after appropriate preoperative staging. Complete resection with systematic mediastinal lymph node evaluation is recommended in this situation, and these patients have improved survival compared with those with N2 disease detected before resection.[1] Adjuvant platinum-based chemotherapy is recommended for these patients based on results from multiple randomized trials and the Lung Adjuvant Cisplatin Evaluation meta-analysis.[2–4] Unresectable N2 disease is defined by bulky, fixed nodes that cannot be individually discerned, are continuous with the primary tumor or encase mediastinal vessels or airways (**Fig. 1**). Numerous prospective trials have clearly demonstrated that adjuvant therapy does not increase resectability and incomplete resection is not associated with a survival benefit.

Resectable or potentially resectable N2 disease is diagnosed during clinical staging and verified by biopsy, but nodes are individually discernible, less than 3 cm, and discrete from the primary tumor (**Fig. 2**). There are multiple treatment strategies for patients with NSCLC with resectable N2 disease,

some of which include surgery and some do not. In the most recent guidelines for lung cancer care from the American College of Chest Physicians, a multidisciplinary approach to potentially resectable N2 disease is recommended.[5] Although upfront resection followed by adjuvant therapy was discouraged in patients with N2 disease identified preoperatively, no recommendation was made regarding definitive chemotherapy and radiation over neoadjuvant therapy and resection. It also notes that there are currently no preoperative factors that can identify which patients benefit from surgery after induction therapy and recommend that the decision to pursue surgery be made before starting induction therapy rather than after.[5] Factors influencing treatment decisions include the size and number of involved nodal stations,[6–8] physiologic status of the patient, and biases of the treating physicians. In 2 independent surveys of thoracic surgeons[9] and medical oncologists[10] regarding treatment practices for N2-positive NSCLC, both groups responded similarly with regard to the central role for resection in the treatment of patients with single-station microscopic N2 disease, but responses diverged with regard to multistation and macroscopic N2 disease. Eighty-two percent of thoracic surgeons compared with only 48% of medical oncologists, saw a role for surgery in multistation macroscopic N2 disease (**Table 1**). The greatest divergence of opinion among surgeons for N2 disease treatment involves those patients who require pneumonectomy, and little consensus currently exists.

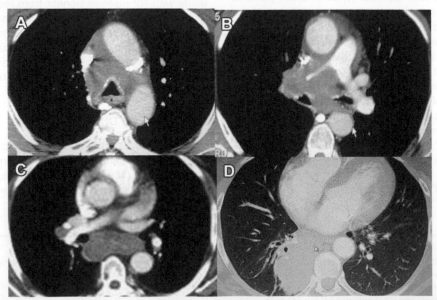

Fig. 1. The CT scans depict unresectable or infiltrative mediastinal lymph node disease due to inability to discern individual nodal stations (*A*), encasement of vessels (*B*), size >3 cm (*C*), and continuity with the primary tumor (*D*).

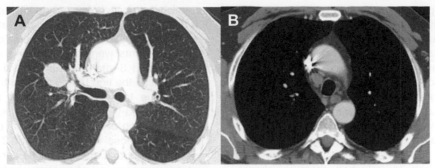

Fig. 2. The CT scan depicts lung windows (*A*) and mediastinal windows (*B*) in a patient with potentially resectable N2 lymph nodes involved with tumor. The lymph nodes are clinically enlarged, but <3 cm, discreet form primary tumor and other nodal stations, and do not encircle or encase mediastinal structures.

The extent of mediastinal lymph node involvement dramatically affects post-resection survival. Andre and colleagues[8] evaluated 700 patients with resected NSCLC, noting that patients with microscopic single-station disease had a 5-year survival similar to that of patients with stage IIB disease at 34%, whereas patients with N2 disease that was clinically evident prior to resection or involvement of multiple stations have 5-year survival rates more closely mirroring stage IIIB at 3-11%. Similarly, a recent large series of incidental and completely resected patients from Ito and colleagues[11] found that the number of N2 nodes (1–2 vs 3–5 vs 6≤), and the rate of N2 involvement amongst resected mediastinal nodes (15%≥ vs 15%–40% vs 40%≤) was prognostic. The location of involved mediastinal nodes also carries prognostic significance. In a series of 141 resected

patients with N2 disease, it was note that patients with left upper lobe tumors involving only aorto-pulmonary lymph nodes had superior survival compared with other N2 patients, and those with lower-lobe tumors metastatic to upper nodal stations and those with upper-lobe tumors metastatic to subcarinal or lower stations had worse prognosis than those with involved nodal stations adjacent to their tumor origin and were not as favorable candidates for resection.[12]

INDUCTION CHEMOTHERAPY

Surgery alone is not a curative treatment option for any patients with N2 disease. Even patients with minimal, single-station, or occult N2 disease have limited survival with surgery alone. Most will eventually relapse systemically. Before 1990,

Table 1
Surgeon and medical oncologist preferences for management of non–small cell lung cancer with N2 involvement

Clinical Scenario	Thoracic Surgeons (n = 513)[9] (%)		Medical Oncologists (n = 406)[10] (%)	
	Role for Surgery	Definitive Chemo/XRT	Role for Surgery	Definitive Chemo/XRT
Single-station, microscopic disease	96	4	92	8
Multistation, macroscopic disease	82	18	48	52
N2 disease and requires R pneumonectomy	30 (pneumonectomy if N2 downstaged) 5 (pneumonectomy regardless of N2 status) 33 (attempt lobectomy if N2 downstaged) 7 (attempt lobectomy only if N2 downstaged)	22	N/R	N/R
Poor PFTs, N2 disease and requires right pneumonectomy	50 (attempt lobectomy)	49	N/R	N/R

Abbreviations: Chemo/XRT, chemotherapy and radiotherapy; N/R, not reported; PFTs, pulmonary function tests.

treatment options were limited in this population, but a series of small phase III trials have since demonstrated a significant survival benefit in patients with stage IIIA NSCLC receiving chemotherapy before resection as compared with resection alone.[13–15] These trials were each quite small and contained many patients not considered IIIA in the current staging system, but the survival differences were significant and induction therapy has become the standard by many for resectable N2 disease. Controversy persists regarding the ideal approach to induction therapy, chemotherapy alone, or concurrent chemotherapy with radiation.

Subsequent phase III trials using induction chemotherapy followed by resection for N2-positive NSCLC have not reported results as impressive as the 3 trials from the early 1990s (**Table 2**). A recent meta-analysis, which included trials outlined in **Table 2**, and 4 additional randomized trials published only in Chinese reported the combined hazard ratio for neoadjuvant chemotherapy for stage IIIA NSCLC was 0.84 (95% confidence interval 0.75–0.95).[16] Many believe that the introduction of third-generation, platinum-based chemotherapy should continue to improve results. These agents produce superior response rates in advanced disease and will likely have a similar impact in the neoadjuvant setting. There is currently a paucity of evidence supporting any one neoadjuvant chemotherapeutic regime over another, but there are shared observations across trials: (1) no significant increase in surgical morbidity or mortality is noted with the addition of induction chemotherapy alone, and (2) the rate of mediastinal nodal clearance is only modest (see **Table 2**).

INDUCTION CHEMORADIOTHERAPY

Trial 8805 from the Southwest Oncology Group (SWOG) was pivotal with regard to our understanding of surgical treatment of stage IIIA NSCLC. It was the first multi-institutional trial to establish feasibility of a trimodality approach to IIIA disease.[17] Patients received cisplatin and etoposide in combination with 4500 cGy of radiation; 85% of patients went on to receive a complete resection and 3-year overall survival was 26%. This was also the first trial to demonstrate a prognostic value for the sterilization of mediastinal lymph nodes; 3-year survival was 44% in patients with eradication of mediastinal nodal disease but only 18% in those with persistent N2 disease at resection. This trial also provided early evidence that pneumonectomy after chemoradiotherapy is associated with an unacceptable increase in toxicity. Mortality following pneumonectomy was 29%.[17] Investigators from the Eastern Cooperative Oncology Group (ECOG) also had reported increased mortality in a very small cohort of patients undergoing pneumonectomy after chemotherapy and 60 Gy of thoracic radiation (43%), but no deaths when the same induction treatment was followed by lobectomy.[18] In this analysis from ECOG, the only factor associated with increased mortality was the use of a pneumonectomy.

Nearly 60% of patients in the SWOG 8805 trial had a complete or near-complete response to induction therapy by pathology after resection. Excellent 5-year survival in these patients caused some to question the additive value of surgery concurrent chemoradiotherapy in N2 positive patients. The North American Intergroup trial 0139 (INT 0139) was designed to address this issue. This phase III trial randomized 396 patients with pathologic N2 disease to cisplatin, etoposide, and concurrent radiation to 45Gy, followed by surgery, or to concurrent chemotherapy and radiation to 61 Gy with out resection. More treatment-related deaths were reported in the trimodality arm (7.9% vs 2.1%), but progression-free survival was longer in that arm: 12.8 versus 10.5 months. Overall survival curves were interesting because they crossed at 2 years, favoring the trimodality arm as time elapsed, with survival of 27.2% compared with 20.3% at 5 years.[19] Pathologic

Table 2
Randomized trials comparing induction chemotherapy alone with surgery

Author, Year	n	% Confirmed N2	Induction Therapy	% 5-y Survival	
				Induction Therapy	Surgery
Roth et al,[13] 1994	60	85	CEP	36	15
Rosell et al,[14] 1994	60	73	MIP	17	9
Depierre et al,[35] 2002	167	N/R	MIP	30	22
Nagai et al,[36] 2003	62	100	PV	23	22

Abbreviations: CEP, cyclophosphamide + etoposide + cisplatin; MIP, mitomycin + ifosfamide + cisplatin; N/R, not reported; PV, vindesine + cisplatin.

eradication of mediastinal lymph node disease was reported in 46%. Five-year survival was improved in this group: 41% compared with only 24% in patients with residual nodal disease. Operative mortality appeared to be clustered in those undergoing resections more extensive than a lobectomy. Mortality was 17.6% for pneumonectomies or complex resections compared with only 1.1% for lobectomy. There was also a very high rate of these extensive resections, with more than one-third of patients receiving a pneumonectomy. An unplanned subset analysis noted important differences in survival based on the extent of resection. Patients undergoing a pneumonectomy did significantly worse than a matched cohort receiving definitive chemoradiation, whereas patients resected by lobectomy did significantly better than a matched cohort that did not undergo resection. The high rate of pneumonectomy paired with the excessive mortality associated with pneumonectomy negatively impacted overall survival in the trimodality arm in this trial. This trial reaffirmed several essential management points with regard to induction therapy and surgery for N2 NSCLC: (1) mediastinal nodal sterilization is a surrogate for improved survival, (2) sterilization rates from this trial are higher than what is reported for chemotherapy alone, (3) 50% of patients have viable tumor in the resected specimen, so surgery is important for local control, and (4) the increased surgical morbidity and mortality appears to be limited to those undergoing pneumonectomy or complex resection.

MORBIDITY AND MORTALITY AFTER INDUCTION THERAPY

The increased operative mortality after induction therapy with both chemotherapy and radiation has been a source of controversy. Although the intergroup trial and SWOG 8805 reported increased complications with a trimodality approach, this is not reported by all. Several single-institution series report acceptable mortality rates for pneumonectomy after induction therapy (0%–13%), with full dose radiation to 60 Gy.[20,21] There is no consensus for stapled versus handsewn bronchial closures, but all recommend autologous soft tissue coverage, meticulous surgical technique, and judicious perioperative fluid administration. Sonett and colleagues[20] also attribute success to the use of 3-dimensional radiation planning, which maximize target doses while sparing surrounding tissue. Despite favorable outcomes, the investigators each stress the importance of using pneumonectomy only as a last resort, and encourage the use of lesser resections and

bronchoplastic procedures when ever possible to still achieve an R0 resection.[20,21]

There is a growing assumption that surgical expertise may be a key component in avoiding morbidity and mortality with a trimodality approach to NSCLC care. Preoperative, intraoperative, and postoperative issues can be challenging and careful patient selection is imperative after induction therapy. The Radiation Therapy Oncology Group (RTOG) has undertaken 2 subsequent trials evaluating trimodality therapy for NSCLC with N2 disease: RTOG 0229 and 0839. Each uses induction radiation dose to 60 Gy in an attempt to increase mediastinal node sterilization, and excluded bulky unresectable mediastinal nodes and tumors that are contiguous with mediastinal nodes. These trials also required surgical certification and incorporated intraoperative and postoperative management requirements in an attempt to decrease operative mortality. Early results of 0229 have been reported with 63% mediastinal nodal clearance and only 1 death in 37 resected patients.[22]

The most worrisome complications following pneumonectomy are postoperative pulmonary edema and bronchopleural fistula. Preoperative thoracic radiotherapy is thought to increase the risk for these complications, due to collateral damage to the residual lung, scarring of mediastinal lymphatics, and reduced vascularity of the bronchial stump. Right pneumonectomies are associated with greater mortality than left pneumonectomies, even in absence of induction therapy.[23] The greater volume of resected lung and decreased arterial vascularization and soft tissue coverage on the right are thought to contribute to the mortality difference. These issues appear to be magnified following thoracic radiation.

MEDIASTINAL RESTAGING

It has become abundantly clear that patients who undergo pathologic downstaging of their mediastinal disease, those that go from cN2 to ypN0, and undergo complete resection have the highest probability for long-term survival. This is the group in which the benefit of resection appears to outweigh the increased risk associated with resection following induction therapy. The difficulty is in accurately identifying these patients preoperatively. Computed tomography (CT) and positron emission tomography (PET) are not currently able do so in the time frame necessary to make clinical decisions. The sensitivity of PET in this setting is only 50% to 60%.[24–26] This means that invasive restaging following induction therapy to establish histologic evidence of downstaging remains an important concern for thoracic surgeons. Repeat mediastinoscopy is performed by some,[27–29] but in general is associated with increased risk for complication and decreased accuracy due to severe adhesions and fibrosis of peritracheal planes.[30] The Cancer and Leukemia Group B (CALGB) recently reported their phase II evaluation of thoracoscopy for restaging of ipsilateral mediastinal nodes. Patients were staged initially by mediastinoscopy and received induction therapy as chemotherapy or radiotherapy alone or in combination. Thoracoscopic restaging was successful in 40%, but unsuccessful in 31%, and incomplete (<3 stations staged) in 29%.[31]

The advent of minimally invasive endobronchial techniques, specifically endobronchial ultrasound (EBUS), with fine-needle aspiration has great potential to impact this surgical challenge. EBUS sensitivity approximates 89% in untreated patients,[32] but unfortunately drops to only 64% following induction therapy.[33] Strategies that use EBUS at initial staging and save mediastinoscopy for restaging after induction treatment would allow for virgin tissue planes and may facilitate safe and accurate postinduction mediastinal node assessment. Establishing accuracy of this approach would represent a tremendous step forward in the surgical management of N2 disease. It would also allow for trials to assess if patients downstaged after induction therapy would have similar survival with or without surgical intervention.

Systematic intra-operative mediastinal lymph node evaluation is strongly recommended in all patients undergoing resection following adjuvant therapy. Persistent mediastinal node disease predicts poor survival and attempt needs to be made to detect this and guide subsequent therapy. There is clinical equipoise between the mediastinal lymph node dissection and systematic sampling in early stage disease,[34] the two approaches have not been formally compared following adjuvant therapy.

T4N2 DISEASE

T4 tumors based on satellite nodules in the same lobe are stage IIIA in the current American Joint Committee on Cancer staging system, and as such are amenable to the treatment plans that include resection. T4 tumors based on extension into the mediastinum, brachial plexus, or spinal structures are considered IIIB when accompanied by N2 nodal involvement. Surgery is typically not recommended for these tumors. These require large and complex resections that are associated with significant morbidity and mortality and are typically reserved for those patients without nodal disease.

SUMMARY

Mediastinal node involvement is the primary determinant for IIIA disease in NSCLC. It is locally advanced disease and curable, but remains a significant treatment challenge. There is no single treatment paradigm appropriate for all patients. The role for surgery is dictated by the ability to perform an R0 resection and by the extent of mediastinal node involvement. For most patients with N2 disease, induction therapy is recommended and survival is closely linked to the response to that treatment. Many believe that a trimodality approach using a combination of chemotherapy, radiation, and surgery provides the best hope for cure, but safety and success is highly dependent on careful patient selection and meticulous treatment delivery.

REFERENCES

1. Cerfolio RJ, Bryant AS. Survival of patients with unsuspected N2 (stage IIIA) nonsmall-cell lung cancer. Ann Thorac Surg 2008;86:362–6 [discussion: 366–7].
2. Douillard JY, Rosell R, De Lena M, et al. Adjuvant vinorelbine plus cisplatin versus observation in patients with completely resected stage IB-IIIA non-small-cell lung cancer (Adjuvant Navelbine International Trialist Association [ANITA]): a randomised controlled trial. Lancet Oncol 2006;7:719–27.
3. Arriagada R, Bergman B, Dunant A, et al. Cisplatin-based adjuvant chemotherapy in patients with completely resected non-small-cell lung cancer. N Engl J Med 2004;350:351–60.
4. Pignon JP, Tribodet H, Scagliotti GV, et al. Lung adjuvant cisplatin evaluation: a pooled analysis by the LACE Collaborative Group. J Clin Oncol 2008; 26:3552–9.
5. Ramnath N, Dilling TJ, Harris LJ, et al. Treatment of stage III non-small cell lung cancer: diagnosis and management of lung cancer, 3rd ed: American College of Chest Physicians evidence-based clinical practice guidelines. Chest 2013;143:e314S–40S.
6. Vansteenkiste JF, De Leyn PR, Deneffe GJ, et al. Clinical prognostic factors in surgically treated stage IIIA-N2 non-small cell lung cancer: analysis of the literature. Lung Cancer 1998;19:3–13.
7. Casali C, Stefani A, Natali P, et al. Prognostic factors in surgically resected N2 non-small cell lung cancer: the importance of patterns of mediastinal lymph nodes metastases. Eur J Cardiothorac Surg 2005;28: 33–8.
8. Andre F, Grunenwald D, Pignon JP, et al. Survival of patients with resected N2 non-small-cell lung cancer: evidence for a subclassification and implications. J Clin Oncol 2000;18:2981–9.

9. Veeramachaneni NK, Feins RH, Stephenson BJ, et al. Management of stage IIIA non-small cell lung cancer by thoracic surgeons in North America. Ann Thorac Surg 2012;94:922–6 [discussion: 926–8].

10. Tanner NT, Gomez M, Rainwater C, et al. Physician preferences for management of patients with stage IIIA NSCLC: impact of bulk of nodal disease on therapy selection. J Thorac Oncol 2012;7:365–9.

11. Ito M, Yamashita Y, Tsutani Y, et al. Classifications of N2 non-small-cell lung cancer based on the number and rate of metastatic mediastinal lymph nodes. Clin Lung Cancer 2013;14:651–7.

12. Okada M, Tsubota N, Yoshimura M, et al. Prognosis of completely resected pN2 non-small cell lung carcinomas: what is the significant node that affects survival? J Thorac Cardiovasc Surg 1999;118: 270–5.

13. Roth JA, Fossella F, Komaki R, et al. A randomized trial comparing perioperative chemotherapy and surgery with surgery alone in resectable stage IIIA non-small-cell lung cancer. J Natl Cancer Inst 1994;86:673–80.

14. Rosell R, Maestre J, Font A, et al. A randomized trial of mitomycin/ifosfamide/cisplatin preoperative chemotherapy plus surgery versus surgery alone in stage IIIA non-small cell lung cancer. Semin Oncol 1994; 21:28–33.

15. Pass HI, Pogrebniak HW, Steinberg SM, et al. Randomized trial of neoadjuvant therapy for lung cancer: interim analysis. Ann Thorac Surg 1992;53: 992–8.

16. Song WA, Zhou NK, Wang W, et al. Survival benefit of neoadjuvant chemotherapy in non-small cell lung cancer: an updated meta-analysis of 13 randomized control trials. J Thorac Oncol 2010;5: 510–6.

17. Albain KS, Rusch VW, Crowley JJ, et al. Concurrent cisplatin/etoposide plus chest radiotherapy followed by surgery for stages IIIA (N2) and IIIB non-small-cell lung cancer: mature results of Southwest Oncology Group phase II study 8805. J Clin Oncol 1995;13:1880–92.

18. Fowler WC, Langer CJ, Curran WJ Jr, et al. Postoperative complications after combined neoadjuvant treatment of lung cancer. Ann Thorac Surg 1993; 55:986–9.

19. Albain KS, Swann RS, Rusch VW, et al. Radiotherapy plus chemotherapy with or without surgical resection for stage III non-small-cell lung cancer: a phase III randomised controlled trial. Lancet 2009; 374:379–86.

20. Sonett JR, Suntharalingam M, Edelman MJ, et al. Pulmonary resection after curative intent radiotherapy (>59 Gy) and concurrent chemotherapy in non-small-cell lung cancer. Ann Thorac Surg 2004; 78:1200–5 [discussion: 1206].

21. Daly BD, Fernando HC, Ketchedjian A, et al. Pneumonectomy after high-dose radiation and concurrent chemotherapy for nonsmall cell lung cancer. Ann Thorac Surg 2006;82:227–31.

22. Suntharalingam M, Paulus R, Edelman MJ, et al. Radiation therapy oncology group protocol 0229: a phase II trial of neoadjuvant therapy with concurrent chemotherapy and full-dose radiation therapy followed by surgical resection and consolidative therapy for locally advanced non-small cell carcinoma of the lung. Int J Radiat Oncol Biol Phys 2012;84: 456–63.

23. Fernandez FG, Force SD, Pickens A, et al. Impact of laterality on early and late survival after pneumonectomy. Ann Thorac Surg 2011;92:244–9.

24. Cerfolio RJ, Ojha B, Mukherjee S, et al. Positron emission tomography scanning with 2-fluoro-2-deoxy-d-glucose as a predictor of response of neoadjuvant treatment for non-small cell carcinoma. J Thorac Cardiovasc Surg 2003;125:938–44.

25. De Leyn P, Stroobants S, De Wever W, et al. Prospective comparative study of integrated positron emission tomography-computed tomography scan compared with remediastinoscopy in the assessment of residual mediastinal lymph node disease after induction chemotherapy for mediastinoscopy-proven stage IIIA-N2 non-small-cell lung cancer: a Leuven Lung Cancer Group Study. J Clin Oncol 2006;24:3333–9.

26. Port JL, Kent MS, Korst RJ, et al. Positron emission tomography scanning poorly predicts response to preoperative chemotherapy in non-small cell lung cancer. Ann Thorac Surg 2004;77:254–9 [discussion: 259].

27. Rami-Porta R, Mateu-Navarro M, Serra-Mitjans M, et al. Remediastinoscopy: comments and updated results. Lung Cancer 2003;42:363–4.

28. Van Schil P, van der Schoot J, Poniewierski J, et al. Remediastinoscopy after neoadjuvant therapy for non-small cell lung cancer. Lung Cancer 2002;37: 281–5.

29. Stamatis G, Fechner S, Hillejan L, et al. Repeat mediastinoscopy as a restaging procedure. Pneumologie 2005;59:862–6.

30. De Waele M, Serra-Mitjans M, Hendriks J, et al. Accuracy and survival of repeat mediastinoscopy after induction therapy for non-small cell lung cancer in a combined series of 104 patients. Eur J Cardiothorac Surg 2008;33:824–8.

31. Jaklitsch MT, Gu L, Demmy T, et al. Prospective phase II trial of preresection thoracoscopic mediastinal restaging after neoadjuvant therapy for IIIA (N2) non-small cell lung cancer: results of CALGB Protocol 39803. J Thorac Cardiovasc Surg 2013; 146:9–16.

32. Silvestri GA, Gonzalez AV, Jantz MA, et al. Methods for staging non-small cell lung cancer: diagnosis

and management of lung cancer, 3rd ed: American College of Chest Physicians evidence-based clinical practice guidelines. Chest 2013;143:e211S–50S.

33. Zielinski M, Szlubowski A, Kolodziej M, et al. Comparison of endobronchial ultrasound and/or endoesophageal ultrasound with transcervical extended mediastinal lymphadenectomy for staging and restaging of non-small-cell lung cancer. J Thorac Oncol 2013;8:630–6.

34. Darling GE, Allen MS, Decker PA, et al. Randomized trial of mediastinal lymph node sampling versus complete lymphadenectomy during pulmonary resection in the patient with N0 or N1 (less than hilar)

non-small cell carcinoma: results of the American College of Surgery Oncology Group Z0030 Trial. J Thorac Cardiovasc Surg 2011;141:662–70.

35. Depierre A, Milleron B, Moro-Sibilot D, et al. Preoperative chemotherapy followed by surgery compared with primary surgery in resectable stage I (except T1N0), II, and IIIa non-small-cell lung cancer. J Clin Oncol 2002;20:247–53.

36. Nagai K, Tsuchiya R, Mori T, et al. A randomized trial comparing induction chemotherapy followed by surgery with surgery alone for patients with stage IIIA N2 non-small cell lung cancer (JCOG 9209). J Thorac Cardiovasc Surg 2003;125:254–60.

Extended Resections of Non-small Cell Lung Cancers Invading the Aorta, Pulmonary Artery, Left Atrium, or Esophagus: Can They Be Justified?

CrossMark

Emily S. Reardon, MD, David S. Schrump, MD, MBA*

KEYWORDS

- Non-small cell lung cancer • T4 • Aorta • Pulmonary artery • Left atrium • Esophagus
- Extended resection

KEY POINTS

- T4 tumors that invade the heart, great vessels, or esophagus comprise a heterogenous group of locally invasive lung cancers.
- Prognosis depends on nodal status.
- Resection should be considered in relation to multidisciplinary care.
- Notable improvements in imaging, surgical techniques, and perioperative care during the past several decades have resulted in an increase in survival for highly selected patients.

INTRODUCTION

Surgical resection remains a critical component of multidisciplinary therapy for locally advanced lung cancers. Non-small cell lung cancers (NSCLC) are highly lethal neoplasms, particularly when diagnosed in advanced stage. More than 50% of NSCLC patients present with metastatic disease or tumors that are unresectable.[1] In stage I NSCLC, for which surgery provides the best chance for cure, overall 5-year survival rates following resection range from 75% to 65% for stage IA and IB tumors, respectively.[2] This rate is in comparison to 5-year survival rates of 24% for stage IIIA and 9% for stage IIIB (T4N2M0) disease.[3] The therapeutic approach for advanced stage NSCLC is controversial, particularly in the surgical management of a subset of T4 tumors invading the heart, great vessels, and other mediastinal structures. However, with modern advances in imaging, surgical techniques, and perioperative care, extended resections may improve survival for highly selected patients.

HISTORICAL BACKGROUND

With the advent of cardiopulmonary bypass (CBP) in the late 1950s, surgeons realized the potential for extracorporeal circulation to facilitate resection of pulmonary malignancies involving the great vessels or atria. In 1965, Neville and colleagues[4] reported a series of 6 patients with lung cancer in whom CPB was used during carinal resection or sleeve lobectomy. One more patient underwent left intrapericardial pneumonectomy with resection and interposition graft repair of the

Disclosures: None.
Thoracic Surgery Section, Thoracic and GI Oncology Branch, CCR/NCI, National Institutes of Health, Building 10, 4-3942, 10 Center Drive, MSC 1201, Bethesda, MD 20892-1201, USA
* Corresponding author. Thoracic and GI Oncology Branch, CCR/NCI, Building 10, 4-3942, 10 Center Drive, MSC 1201, Bethesda, MD 20892-1201.
E-mail address: david.schrump@nih.gov

Thorac Surg Clin 24 (2014) 457–464
http://dx.doi.org/10.1016/j.thorsurg.2014.07.012
1547-4127/14/$ – see front matter Published by Elsevier Inc.

descending aorta. Disappointingly, 6 of the 7 patients died in the immediate postoperative period from bleeding, heart failure, or pulmonary edema. Several years later, Bailey and colleagues[5] described 2 patients with lung cancer in whom CPB was used to facilitate extended left pneumonectomy. The first patient required left intrapericardial pneumonectomy with en bloc resection and direct suture repair of the left atrium as well as resection and interposition graft repair of the descending aorta. The second patient underwent left intrapericardial pneumonectomy, resection and repair of the left atrium, and resection and repair of the distal main pulmonary artery. Both patients were fully heparinized and cannulated for venous return via the main pulmonary artery, and arterial inflow by 2 sites in the aorta, proximal and distal to the lines of surgical resection. The first patient developed coagulopathy and died in the early postoperative period. The second patient, whose pathologic stage by description was T4N1, survived 14 months before succumbing to metastatic disease. Although sophisticated staging systems and prognostic indicators for lung cancer had not yet been developed, the aforementioned authors understood the principles of en bloc tumor resection with minimal manipulation, the significance of tumor histology and mediastinal lymph node metastases, and the consequences of coagulopathy complicating pneumonectomy.

MORE RECENT EXPERIENCE

The value of surgical resection for the treatment of T4 NSCLCs invading the aorta, pulmonary artery, left atrium, and esophagus remains open to debate. Presently, most patients are not offered resection in part because of the potential for significant morbidity and mortality. However, perioperative risk in this subset of patients has improved over time (**Table 1**). In 1987, Burt and colleagues[6] published a retrospective review of 225 patients who underwent thoracotomy for primary NSCLC invading the mediastinum. Lesions were classified as T3, "a tumor of any size with direct extension into an adjacent structure such as the mediastinum and its contents," according to TNM descriptors used by the Union for International

Table 1
Selected summary of extended resections of T4 NSCLC

Reference	T4 Sites of Disease	Patients	Morbidity (%)	Mortality (%)	Overall Survival (% at 5 y)
Burt et al,[6] 1987	Aorta, pulmonary artery, esophagus	225	NR	2.7	9
Tsuchiya et al,[7] 1994	Aorta, left atrium, pulmonary artery, SVC	101	NR	NR	13
Martini et al,[8] 1994	Aorta, left atrium, pulmonary artery, SVC, esophagus, trachea, spine	102	NR	6	19
Bernard et al,[9] 2001	Aorta, left atrium, pulmonary artery, SVC, esophagus, carina, spine	77	NR	NR	21[a]
Pitz et al,[10] 2003	Aorta, left atrium, pulmonary artery, SVC, esophagus, trachea, carina, spine	89	NR	19	19
Ratto et al,[11] 2004	Left atrium	19	37	0	14
Ohta et al,[12] 2005	Aorta	16	31	12.5	48
Yildizeli et al,[13] 2008	Aorta, left atrium, pulmonary artery, SVC, esophagus, carina, spine, subclavian artery/vein, carotid artery, chest wall	271	35	4	38
Wu et al,[14] 2009	Left atrium	46	52	0	22
Yang et al,[15] 2009	Aorta, left atrium, pulmonary artery, SVC, esophagus, trachea, carina, spine	146	53	3.1	23
Spaggiari et al,[16] 2013	Aorta, left atrium, SVC, carina	167	34	5	23
Galvaing et al,[17] 2014	Left atrium	19	53	11	44

Abbreviation: NR, not recorded.
[a] Survival rate at 3 years.

Cancer Control in the early 1980s. This classification included tumors that invaded adjacent organs.[18,19] Approximately 10% of patients with mediastinal invasion had aorta involvement, one-third of whom had simultaneous involvement of the pulmonary artery.[6] Most of these patients also had mediastinal lymph node metastases. They observed a superior perioperative mortality of 2.7%, and a nonfatal complication rate of 13%. Complete (R0) resection was associated with a survival advantage, with a median survival of 17 months and 5-year survival of 9%. In 1989, Nakahara and colleagues[20] reported successful en bloc pulmonary and aortic resection in 3 patients with lung cancer with the use of CPB, one of whom was alive 17 months following surgery.

In 1994, Tsuchiya and colleagues[7] summarized the results of en bloc lung and aortic resection as a portion of a larger clinical series involving T4 tumors. Twenty-one patients with aortic involvement had dissection in a subadventitial plane. Resection was thought to be incomplete in 12 of these patients. Seven patients with aortic involvement (6 with invasion near the ligamentum arteriosum, 1 with subclavian artery involvement) underwent complete resection. Two patients received graft replacement using subclavian artery to descending aorta bypass. An additional 7 patients underwent resection of the main pulmonary artery using full CPB support. Not surprisingly, multivariate analysis revealed that survival depended on perioperative bleeding, postoperative pneumonia, completeness of resection, and nodal status. Pathologic staging and survival for these patients undergoing aortic resection were not documented clearly in the publication. However, it was noted that one of the patients was alive 9 years following the operation. In that same year, Martini and colleagues[8] also described 102 patients with NSCLC invading the mediastinum, excluding those who had N2 disease. In this study, patients were divided into subgroups based on extent of mediastinal invasion and classified as T3 or T4. Forty-four of the patients had T4 tumors that invaded the aorta, superior vena cava (SVC), esophagus, trachea, spine, or atrium. Overall, operative mortality was 6% and 5-year survival was 19%. With complete resection, 5-year survival was 30%.

In response to the emerging controversy surrounding extended resections of T4 NSCLC, multiple retrospective studies were published providing additional data to support the concept that properly selected patients could benefit from the procedure.[21] These observational studies attempted to identify those patients who were more likely to benefit from extended resection within a heterogeneous population of T4 tumors.

In 2001, Bernard and colleagues[9] conducted a retrospective cohort study of 77 patients with T4 NSCLCs that invaded the mediastinum by direct extension or comprised multiple synchronous lesions within the same lobe of the lung, the latter of which are now classified as T3 lesions.[1] One-year and 5-year survival rates were 33% and 0% for 8 patients with aortic invasion, 40% and 8% for 19 patients with left atrial invasion, and 20% and 12% for 8 patients with esophageal invasion. Nodal status (pN0 or pN1 vs pN2) was associated with survival. Improved 5-year survival rates were also described in retrospective studies of extended resection of T4 NSCLCs with mediastinal involvement alone. Wu and colleagues[14] and Yang and colleagues[15] reported 5-year overall survival rates of 22% and 23%, respectively. In 2003, Pitz and colleagues[10] noted an improved 5-year survival rate of 46% following R0 resection of T4 tumors with invasion of major mediastinal structures, including the aorta, pulmonary artery, left atrium, and esophagus. Nevertheless, this was also associated with significant hospital mortality (19%). Similarly, in 2 retrospective reviews by Mu and colleagues[22] and Wang and colleagues,[23] each involving more than 100 patients, overall 5-year survival rates of 43% and 41% were observed in T4 NSCLCs invading the left atrium and great vessels. Operative morbidity and mortality were not reported for these series.

In a retrospective cohort study using the SEER database, Farjah and colleagues[24] examined trends in the operative management and outcomes of patients with T4 lung cancers treated between 1992 and 2002 in the United States. A total of 13,077 patients with stage IIIB disease defined by T4 tumors were identified, of which only 9% underwent resection. The specific locations of the T4 tumors were not evaluated. Thirty-day mortality was 10% and this did not change significantly over time. Factors associated with higher odds of operative mortality included increasing age, CCI (Klabunde-modified Charlson Comorbidity Index)[25] higher than 0, tumor size 3 cm or larger, or pneumonectomy. Five-year overall survival and lung cancer cause-specific survival did increase over time from 15% to 35% and 33% to 50%, respectively. The authors concluded that the temporal changes observed in the operative management of T4 tumors coincided with improvements in long-term survival, and that these findings supported resection for select patients with these neoplasms.

Superior outcomes are particularly evident when extended resections are performed at high-volume, specialized institutions where surgical techniques and perioperative care have been refined. In 2008, Yildizeli and colleagues[13] published an institutional review representing 25 years of experience in radical surgery for clinically staged T4 N0/N1 NSCLC. Of 271 patients with tumors involving the carina, SVC, mediastinum, heart, and great vessels, overall rates of 30-day mortality and morbidity were 4% and 35%, respectively. Patients were divided into 4 subgroups: superior sulcus tumors (n = 126); carinal invasion (n = 92); SVC invasion (n = 39); and mediastinal (n = 14), including tumors that invaded the aorta (n = 2), pulmonary artery (n = 3), left atrium (n = 7), and esophagus (n = 2). A total of 11 patients died postoperatively, of which 6 had bronchopleural fistulas. Organ-specific rates of mortality were listed for invasion of the aorta (14%), right or left pulmonary artery (21%), left atrium (50%), and esophagus (14%). Notably, only 9 operations were performed using CPB. The most common complications were pulmonary edema and atelectasis. Median length of hospitalization was 15 days. Overall 5-year and 10-year survivals were 36.6% and 25.9%, respectively, with a median survival of 28 months. Five-year survival for the mediastinal group alone was 61%. Multivariate analysis demonstrated that 3 factors independently influenced survival: nodal status (N0/N1 vs N2/N3/M1), complete resection (R0 vs R1; 40.4% vs 15.9%), and noninvasion of the subclavian artery. Likewise, in 2013, Spaggiari and colleagues[16] reported survival after extended resection for 167 cases of lung cancers invading mediastinal structures. They observed an overall morbidity of 34% and postoperative mortality of 5% at 30 days and 11% at 90 days. Overall 5-year survival data according to nearby organ invasion were also documented, which demonstrated a trend toward better long-term survival in patients with aorta invasion. Organ-specific postoperative complications were not reported in this study. Five-year survival rates were aorta (37%), left atrium (25%), carina (22%), and SVC (26%). Factors that positively influenced survival included R0 resection and pN0 disease.

EXTENDED RESECTIONS
Aorta

If there is no evidence of intrapleural dissemination or mediastinal nodal involvement, and there is direct tumor invasion of the aorta, en bloc pulmonary and aortic resection can be considered. Of particular note is the fixation of the tumor to the distal arch and proximal descending aorta, which limits one's ability to manipulate the hilum. The extent of the tumor within the lung dictates whether lobectomy or pneumonectomy is necessary. The arch of the aorta is mobilized and control of the left subclavian and distal arch is obtained. Although historically, aortic resections have been performed using left heart bypass, some centers use clamp-and-sew techniques or passive shunts without bypass.[13,15,16,26]

Several studies have demonstrated that long-term survival is possible with resection of the aorta en bloc with primary tumor (see **Table 1**).[7–10,12,13,15,16,20,26–30] In general, when compared with other mediastinal structures, resection of the aorta has been associated with a higher operative morbidity and mortality, and this seems to correlate with the use of CPB. In 2005, Ohta and colleagues[12] published a series of 16 patients who underwent thoracic aorta resection along with left pneumonectomy (n = 6), left upper lobectomy (n = 9), and partial lung resection (n = 1) with the use of CPB in 10 patients, and a passive shunt between the ascending and descending aorta in 4 patients. Postoperative mortality was 12.5% and morbidity was 31%, with 6 major complications occurring in 5 patients. Four patients suffered significant postoperative bleeding. Three patients had intrapleural bleeding and one died from this event. One patient died of severe hemorrhage following an aortic laceration just distal to the left subclavian artery. Twelve (75%) patients had complete resection. Median survival time for all patients was 26 months, with a 5-year survival rate of 48.2%, and median and 5-year survival rates for patients with pathologic N0 disease were 31 months and 70%, respectively.

Other studies, which have included patients with resection of T4 NSCLCs invading the aorta, have also demonstrated improved long-term survival but have not reported their respective rates of morbidity or mortality. In a retrospective review of 13 patients with T4 tumors requiring aorta resection without the use of CPB, Misthos and colleagues[26] reported a 5-year survival of 31%; associated postoperative complications and mortality were not documented. Similarly, in the recent review published by Spaggiari and colleagues,[16] no extracorporeal circulation was used for the 14 patients requiring aorta resection. These authors noted a 5-year overall survival for patients with aorta invasion of 37%. Overall morbidity and 30-day mortality were 34% and 5%, respectively. Organ-specific complication rates were not recorded.

Pulmonary Artery

Resection and reconstruction of the pulmonary artery in patients with lung cancer is technically feasible. The procedure is usually indicated for tumors or satellite lymph nodes that involve the pulmonary artery at the hilum and preclude resection by simple lobectomy. The extent of involvement varies, from partial infiltration to more extensive and circumferential invasion.[31] Early reports describing the technique were associated with significant mortality and poor overall survival, where all postoperative survivors died soon after resection from recurrent cancer.[7–9,29,31–34]

To address the safety and long-term outcome for reconstruction of the pulmonary artery, Venuta and colleagues[31] recently reported their 20-year experience and demonstrated improved outcomes. On review of data gathered from 1989 to 2008, of 105 patients, overall morbidity was 28.5%. Two major complications were noted: one pulmonary artery thrombosis, requiring completion pneumonectomy on postoperative day 2, and one massive hemoptysis leading to death in a patient who had undergone combined bronchovascular reconstruction. Of note, not all the patients evaluated had T4 tumors with invasion of the pulmonary artery. Only 22% were classified as stage IIIB, and the extent of tumor involvement was not documented. Operative mortality was 0.95%, and overall 5-year and 10-year survivals were 44% and 20%, respectively. As expected, nodal status had a significant effect on survival. Patients with N0 disease had 5-year and 10-year survival rates of 67% and 33%, compared with 20% and 3%, respectively, for patients with N2 disease. Reconstruction involved patch reconstruction (n = 55), end-to-end anastomosis (n = 47), or interposition with use of a prosthetic conduit (n = 3). In 65 patients (62%), pulmonary artery reconstruction was performed along with bronchial sleeve resection, and in all other cases, either standard lobectomy or bilobectomy was performed. More recently, Berthet and colleagues[35] published their single institutional experience of 178 patients with centrally located NSCLC requiring resection of the pulmonary artery, and reconstruction or replacement, with or without concomitant sleeve bronchial resection. Although safety and efficacy of the procedure can be fairly assessed, a limited number of patients in this study had T4 tumors (n = 1), and therefore, comparisons of overall survival cannot be made. Pulmonary artery reconstruction was performed in 32 (35%) patients (2 by autologous pericardium patch and 20 by end-to-end anastomosis). Pulmonary artery replacement was performed in the remaining cases primarily with the use of cryopreserved arterial allograft (aortic allograft was used in 3 patients). R0 resection was achieved in all patients. There were no hospital deaths. Four major and 2 minor postoperative complications were reported, including one allograft thrombosis.

Mu and colleagues[22] and Wang and colleagues[23] have each retrospectively analyzed their survival data following resection of T4 NSCLCs that invade the great vessels and left atrium. Neither study documents postoperative complications. In the study by Mu and colleagues,[22] 136 patients required resection of the pulmonary artery (n = 83), SVC (n = 21), or left atrium (n = 32). Five-year overall survival was 43% for all patients and 53% in the pulmonary artery group. Wang and colleagues[23] evaluated 105 patients with tumors invading the pulmonary artery (n = 57), SVC (n = 23), and left atrium (n = 25). They demonstrated similar survival rates, in which 5-year survival for all patients was 41%. In those patients undergoing pulmonary artery resection, 5-year survival was 46% and median survival was approximately 50 months.

Left Atrium

NSCLC can involve the left atrium either via direct invasion or by tumor embolus into the pulmonary vein. Many of the original reports describing resection of tumors involving adjacent mediastinal structures included patients with left atrial involvement, but the extent of atrial wall invasion was unclear.[6–9,21,30,34] Macchiarini and Dartevelle[36] reported that in 31 patients, 17 with direct invasion and 13 with tumor embolization, resection was associated with a 22% 5-year survival. However, all patients with embolic left atrial disease died of distant hematogenous metastasis with a median disease-free interval of only 6 months.[32]

In 2004 and 2005, 2 retrospective reviews were published detailing single-institution experiences in the surgical management of T4 lesions invading the left atrium. Ratto and colleagues[11] reported 19 patients with T4 lesions invading the left atrial wall. Atrial resection was performed by applying a vascular clamp to the left atrium, at times dissecting the interatrial septum for adequate tumor resection and directly suturing the defect. Pneumonectomy was performed in 12 patients and lobectomy was performed in 7 patients. Complete resection was achieved in 11 patients (58%), but a significant percentage (58%) had pathologic N2 disease. Morbidity and mortality were 37% and 0%, respectively. Six patients experienced postoperative arrhythmia, and one had a cerebrovascular accident. Median survival was 25 months, and 5-year survival was 14%. Spaggiari and colleagues[37] reported 15 patients who underwent extended pneumonectomy with partial resection of the left atrium. The authors describe a more homogenous population and surgical approach involving intrapericardial pneumonectomy with resection of the left atrium and dissection along the groove of Sondergaard in an effort to increase the margin of resection. All patients had R0 resections. Morbidity was 15.3% with no major postoperative complications, and mortality was 0%. Long-term survival was not reported; median follow-up was 16.5 months. At the completion of the study, 9 patients (60%) were still alive, of whom 8 had no evidence of disease. In a subsequent publication pertaining to 167 patients with T4 tumors, including 35 patients who underwent left atrial resection between 1998 and 2010, Spaggiari and colleagues[16] reported an overall 5-year survival rate of 27%. Mu and colleagues[22] and Wang and colleagues[23] published similar results; respective 5-year survival rates for patients requiring left atrial resection were 18% (n = 32) and 36% (n = 25).

More recently, Galvaing and colleagues[17] published their results of 19 patients who underwent left atrial resection for T4 lung cancer between the years 2004 and 2012. In all patients, left atrial invasion was suspected preoperatively. Cardiac MRI was obtained to assess for the extent of invasion; none had suspected invasion of both atria, the presence of an intra-atrial thrombi, or polypoid tumor inside the atrium. Patients were classified according to the extent of dissection along the interatrial septum, with most of the dissection involving sectioning of the interatrial muscle. The authors report an R0 resection in 17 patients and R1 resection in the remaining 3 patients. Similar to previous reports, a significant number of patients had pN2 disease (37%). Overall postoperative morbidity was 53% (n = 10) and operative mortality was 11% (n = 2). The 5-year survival rate was 44%. The recurrence rate was 21%; 2 patients had distant disease and 2 patients had local disease at the time of recurrence. Interestingly, 3 patients were alive for greater than 6 years postoperatively.

Esophagus

Involvement of the esophagus by direct extension of primary lung cancer is rare. However, local invasion has been reported and is typically limited to excision of the muscular wall.[6,8–10,13–16,21–24,27,29,33,38] Associated morbidity, mortality, and long-term survival are therefore difficult to quantify. In a univariate analysis of survival rates according to T4 sites of mediastinal involvement, of 8 patients with esophageal resection, one patient survived 5 years.[9]

PREOPERATIVE WORKUP

The principles of en bloc pulmonary and mediastinal excision for T4 lung cancer must follow a well-defined algorithm during which the patient is thoroughly staged preoperatively and intraoperatively before definitive resection. Criteria should include appropriate pulmonary reserve for pneumonectomy, if indicated, and no evidence of mediastinal nodal or distant metastatic disease. Although incapable of definitively documenting aortic invasion by tumor, cardiac MR scans have emerged as highly useful adjuncts for delineating extent of tumor involvement in the mediastinum. Transesophageal echocardiography can also be used to detect left atrial invasion as well as to assess the extent of atherosclerotic disease in the distal aortic arch and proximal descending aorta, which could complicate resection. Histologically normal mucosa must be documented at the site of intended resection, and comprehensive mediastinoscopy should be performed to evaluate subcarinal and contralateral paratracheal nodal stations. Any evidence of contralateral mediastinal nodal disease is an absolute contraindication to extended resection because expected median survival in patients with N3 disease is only 12 months[39] and the benefits of extended resections for patients with ipsilateral N2 involvement are limited at best. If no evidence of nodal disease is detected by mediastinoscopy, one can then proceed directly to thoracotomy or sternotomy to assess resectability and biopsy additional nodal stations not accessible by this technique. Thoracoscopic staging is a possible alternative modality. However, an open procedure minimizes intraoperative time and provides maximal opportunity to thoroughly evaluate all nodal stations. In their analysis of trends in the management and outcomes of T4 lung cancers from 1998 to 2002, Farjah and colleagues[24] reported a high proportion (22%) of pN2/N3 disease. The authors suggest that this may be correlated with infrequent use of both PET and mediastinoscopy (10% in the year 2002), advocating for the use of a more extensive preoperative workup to better select patients with N0-1 disease.

NEOADJUVANT THERAPY

The use of neoadjuvant therapy to achieve the goals of down-staging locally advanced lung cancers, by reducing tumor size and lymph node involvement, and potentially eradicating micrometastatic disease, can be applied to T4 tumors with invasion of the aorta, pulmonary artery, left atrium, or esophagus. Induction therapy used for this subset of T4 tumors is an extension of stage IIIA (N2) preoperative chemotherapy or chemoradiotherapy, which is still heavily debated.[40–43] To date, induction therapy followed by extended resection for this small subset of T4 tumors has been disparately used, with very little data to provide meaningful recommendations.

SUMMARY

T4 tumors that invade the heart, great vessels, or esophagus comprise a heterogenous group of locally invasive lung cancers. Prognosis depends on nodal status; this relationship has been consistently demonstrated in many of the small series of extended resection. Current National Comprehensive Cancer Network guidelines do not recommend surgery for T4 extension with N2-3 disease (stage IIIB). However, biopsy-proven T4 N0-1 (stage IIIA) may be operable.[1] Localized tumors with invasion of the aorta, pulmonary artery, left atrium, or esophagus represent a small subset of T4 disease. Acquiring sufficient randomized data to provide statistical proof of a survival advantage for patients undergoing extended resections for these neoplasms will likely never be possible. Therefore, we are left to critically analyze current documented experience to make clinical decisions on a case-by-case basis.

It is clear that the operative morbidity and mortality of extended resections for locally advanced T4 tumors have significantly improved over time, yet the risks are still high. The indications for such procedures and the anticipated outcomes should be clearly weighed in terms of potential perioperative complications and expertise of the surgical team. Patients with T4 N0-1 have the best prognosis and with complete resection may have the potential for cure. The use of induction therapy and surgery for advanced T4 tumors may improve survival. Current data suggest that for tumors that invade the aorta, pulmonary artery, left atrium, or esophagus, resection should be considered in relation to multidisciplinary care. For properly selected patients receiving treatment at high volume, experienced centers, extended resections may be warranted.

REFERENCES

1. Ettinger DS, Wood, DE, Akerley W, et al. NCCN clinical practice guidelines in oncology: non-small cell lung cancer. Version 2.2014. Available at: http://www.nccn.org/professionals/physician_gls/pdf/nscl.pdf.
2. Kassis ES, Vaporciyan AA, Swisher SG, et al. Application of the revised lung cancer staging system (IASLC Staging Project) to a cancer center population. J Thorac Cardiovasc Surg 2009;138(2):412–8.
3. Goldstraw P, Crowley J, Chansky K, et al. The IASLC lung cancer staging project: proposals for the revision of the TNM stage groupings in the forthcoming (seventh) edition of the TNM classification of malignant tumours. J Thorac Oncol 2007;2(8):706–14.
4. Neville WE, Langston HT, Correll N, et al. Cardiopulmonary bypass during pulmonary surgery. J Thorac Cardiovasc Surg 1965;50:265–76.
5. Bailey CP, Schechter DC, Folk FS. Extending operability in lung cancer involving the heart and great vessels. Ann Thorac Surg 1971;11(2):140–50.
6. Burt ME, Pomerantz AH, Bains MS, et al. Results of surgical treatment of stage III lung cancer invading the mediastinum. Surg Clin North Am 1987;67(5):987–1000.
7. Tsuchiya R, Asamura H, Kondo H, et al. Extended resection of the left atrium, great vessels, or both for lung cancer. Ann Thorac Surg 1994;57(4):960–5.
8. Martini N, Yellin A, Ginsberg RJ, et al. Management of non-small cell lung cancer with direct mediastinal involvement. Ann Thorac Surg 1994;58(5):1447–51.
9. Bernard A, Bouchot O, Hagry O, et al. Risk analysis and long-term survival in patients undergoing resection of T4 lung cancer. Eur J Cardiothorac Surg 2001;20(2):344–9.
10. Pitz C, de la Riviere A, van Swieten H, et al. Results of surgical treatment of T4 non-small cell lung cancer. Eur J Cardiothorac Surg 2003;24:1013–8.
11. Ratto GB, Costa R, Vassallo G, et al. Twelve-year experience with left atrial resection in the treatment of non-small cell lung cancer. Ann Thorac Surg 2004;78(1):234–7.
12. Ohta M, Hirabayasi H, Shiono H, et al. Surgical resection for lung cancer with infiltration of the thoracic aorta. J Thorac Cardiovasc Surg 2005;129(4):804–8.
13. Yildizeli B, Dartevelle PG, Fadel E, et al. Results of primary surgery with T4 non-small cell lung cancer during a 25-year period in a single center: the benefit is worth the risk. Ann Thorac Surg 2008;86(4):1065–75.
14. Wu L, Zhifei X, Zhao X, et al. Surgical treatment of lung cancer invading the left atrium or base of the pulmonary vein. World J Surg 2009;33:492–6.
15. Yang H, Hou X, Lin P, et al. Survival and risk factors of surgically treated mediastinal invasion T4 non-small cell lung cancer. Ann Thorac Surg 2009;88:372–9.
16. Spaggiari L, Tessitore A, Casiraghi M, et al. Survival after extended resection for mediastinal advanced lung cancer: lessons learned on 167 consecutive cases. Ann Thorac Surg 2013;95:117–25.
17. Galvaing G, Tardy M, Cassagnes L, et al. Left atrial resection for T4 lung cancer without cardiopulmonary

bypass: technical aspects and outcomes. Ann Thorac Surg 2014;97(5):1708–13.

18. Mountain CF, Carr DT, Anderson WA. A system for the clinical staging of lung cancer. Am J Roentgenol Radium Ther Nucl Med 1974;120:130–8.

19. Goldstraw P. New staging system: how does it affect our practice? J Clin Oncol 2013;31(8):984–91.

20. Nakahara K, Ohno K, Mastumura A, et al. Extended operation for lung cancer invading the aortic arch and superior vena cava. J Thorac Cardiovasc Surg 1989;97(3):428–33.

21. Chambers A, Routledge T, Bille A, et al. Does surgery have a role in T4N0 and T4N1 lung cancer? Interact Cardiovasc Thorac Surg 2010;11:473–9.

22. Mu JW, Wang YG, Li J, et al. Surgical results of T4 lung cancer invading left atrium and great vessels. Zhonghua Yi Xue Za Zhi 2008;88(6):383–6.

23. Wang X, Liu T, Yin X. Surgical treatment of IIIb-T4 lung cancer invading left atrium and great vessels. Chin Med J 2010;123(3):365–8.

24. Farjah F, Wood DE, Varghese TK, et al. Trends in the operative management and outcomes of T4 lung cancer. Ann Thorac Surg 2008;86:368075.

25. Klabunde CN, Potosky AL, Legler JM, et al. Development of a comorbidity index using physician claims data. J Clin Epidemiol 2000;53:1258–67.

26. Misthos P, Papagiannakis G, Kokotsakis J, et al. Surgical management of lung cancer invading the aorta or the superior vena cava. Lung Cancer 2007;56: 223–7.

27. Klepetko W, Wisser W, Birsan T, et al. T4 lung tumors with infiltration of the thoracic aorta: is an operation reasonable? Ann Thorac Surg 1999;67(2):340–4.

28. De Perrot M, Fadel E, Mussot S, et al. Resection of locally advanced (T4) non-small cell lung cancer with cardiopulmonary bypass. Ann Thorac Surg 2005;79(5):1961–7.

29. Shiraishi T, Shirakusa T, Miyoshi T, et al. Extended resection of T4 lung cancer with invasion of the aorta: is it justified? Thorac Cardiovasc Surg 2005; 53(6):375–9.

30. Kauffmann M, Kruger T, Aebert H. Surgery on extracorporeal circulation in early and advanced nonsmall cell lung cancer. Thorac Cardiovasc Surg 2013;61(2):103–8.

31. Venuta F, Ciccone AM, Anile M, et al. Reconstruction of the pulmonary artery for lung cancer: long-term results. J Thorac Cardiovasc Surg 2009;138(5):1185–91.

32. Rice TW, Blackstone EH. Radical resections for T4 lung cancer. Surg Clin North Am 2002;82(3):573–87.

33. Izbicki JR, Knoefel WT, Passlick B, et al. Risk analysis and long-term survival in patients undergoing extended resection of locally advanced lung cancer. J Thorac Cardiovasc Surg 1995;110(2):386–95.

34. Fukuse T, Wada H, Hitomi S, et al. Extended resection of the left atrium, great vessels, or both for lung cancer. Eur J Cardiothorac Surg 1997;11(4): 664–9.

35. Berthet JP, Boada M, Paradela M, et al. Pulmonary sleeve resection in locally advanced lung cancer using cryopreserved allograft for pulmonary artery replacement. J Thorac Cardiovasc Surg 2013;146: 1191–7.

36. Macchiarini P, Dartevelle P. Extended resections for lung cancer. In: Roth JA, Cox JD, Hong WK, editors. Lung cancer. 2nd edition. Malden (MA): Blackwell Science Inc; 1998. p. 135–61.

37. Spaggiari L, D'Aiuto M, Veronesi G, et al. Extended pneumonectomy with partial resection of the left atrium, without cardiopulmonary bypass, for lung cancer. Ann Thorac Surg 2005;79(1):234–40.

38. Bryant A, Pereira S, Miller D, et al. Satellite pulmonary nodule in the same lobe (T4N0) should not be staged as IIIB non-small cell lung cancer. Ann Thorac Surg 2006;82:1808–14.

39. Rusch VW, Crowley J, Giroux DJ, et al. The IASLC Lung Cancer Staging Project: proposals for the revision of the N descriptors in the forthcoming seventh edition of the TNM Classification for lung cancer. J Thorac Oncol 2007;2(7):603–12.

40. Martins RG, D'Amico TA, Loo BW Jr, et al. The management of patients with stage IIIA non-small cell lung cancer with N2 mediastinal node involvement. J Natl Compr Canc Netw 2012;10(5):599–613.

41. Albain K, Swann RS, Rusch VW, et al. Radiotherapy plus chemotherapy with or without surgical resection for stage III non-small cell lung cancer: a phase III randomized control trial. Lancet 2009;374(9687): 379–86.

42. van Meerbeeck JP, Kramer GW, Van Schil PE, et al. Randomized controlled trial of resection versus radiotherapy after induction chemotherapy in stage IIIA-N2 non-small cell lung cancer. J Natl Cancer Inst 2007;99(6):442–50.

43. Schrump DS, Carter D, Kelsey CR, et al. "Non-Small Cell Lung Cancer". In: DeVita VT, Lawrence TS, Rosenberg SA, editors. Cancer: principles and practice of oncology. 9th edition. Philadelphia: Lippincott Williams & Wilkins; 2011. p. 799–847. Print.

Video-Assisted Thoracoscopic (VATS) Lobectomy After Induction Therapy

Nathan M. Mollberg, DO, Michael S. Mulligan, MD*

KEYWORDS

• Lobectomy • Induction therapy • Video-assisted thoracoscopic surgery • VATS • Neoadjuvant

KEY POINTS

- As experience with video-assisted thoracoscopic lobectomy has increased, its application toward more technically demanding operations has expanded to surgical treatment after induction therapy in select patients.
- This approach is designed for maximal safety and has been used with great success on patients who have undergone induction therapy.
- The demand for precision is far greater in these cases and the tempo of dissection should be slowed.

INTRODUCTION

Neoadjuvant chemotherapy or chemoradiotherapy is largely reserved for advanced-stage lung cancers. Increased rates of major morbidity and mortality were reported in early experiences with open lobectomy after neoadjuvant chemoradiotherapy.[1] However, more recent reports have shown similar early outcomes compared with surgery alone.[2] Concerns regarding the sequelae of neoadjuvant chemotherapy or chemoradiotherapy on the pleural space and tissue planes had previously deterred the application of video-assisted thoracoscopic (VATS) lobectomy for patients who underwent neoadjuvant therapy. As experience with VATS has increased, however, its application toward more technically demanding operations has also expanded. Nonrandomized studies comparing open lobectomy and VATS have shown shorter length of hospitalization and chest tube duration, decreased postoperative pain, lower complication rates, and shorter recovery time for patients undergoing VATS. In addition, multiple reports have demonstrated oncologic equivalence with open thoracotomy. Therefore, the motive to apply a minimally invasive approach to lung resection after neoadjuvant therapy would be to decrease patient discomfort and length of stay without sacrificing oncologic efficacy.

OUTCOMES

The largest series reported to date is from the First Affiliated Hospital of Guangzhou Medical University in China (**Table 1**). Huang and colleagues[3] retrospectively reviewed 43 patients who underwent induction therapy (27 received chemotherapy alone whereas 16 received chemoradiation) followed by VATS resection. Although 33 (77%) patients underwent lobectomy or bilobectomy, the authors included 5 (12%) patients who underwent wedge resection and 4 (9%) who underwent pneumonectomy in their analysis. Most patients (63%) had clinical stage IIIA disease. Patients

The authors have nothing to disclose.
Division of Cardiothoracic Surgery, Department of Surgery, University of Washington, Seattle, WA 98195, USA
* Corresponding author. University of Washington Medical Center, 1959 Northeast Pacific Street, Box 356310, Seattle, WA 98195-6310.
E-mail address: msmmd@u.washington.edu

Table 1
Neoadjuvant therapy outcomes in recent research

Reference	Study Design	n	Type of Neoadjuvant Therapy	Conversion to Thoracotomy (%)	Stage ≥III (%)	Morbidity (%)	Mortality (%)
Huang et al,[3] 2013	Retrospective	43	5 (12%) gefitinib; 38 (88%) platinum-based chemotherapy; 13 (30%) concurrent radiotherapy; 3 (7%) sequential radiotherapy	16	88	12	2
Petersen et al,[4] 2006	Retrospective	12	11 (92%) platinum-based chemotherapy; 8 (76%) concurrent radiotherapy	8	75	8	0
Shaw et al,[5] 2008	Retrospective	10	10 (100%) platinum-based chemotherapy with concurrent radiotherapy	Not reported	100	30	0

who underwent neoadjuvant radiotherapy received a dose of 40 Gy. Although the authors reported overall complication and mortality rates of 12% and 2%, respectively, these were not stratified by extent of resection or type of induction therapy. Reporting on conversion to thoracotomy was also unclear, because 1 patient was reported to have not undergone VATS and an additional 7 (16%) were stated to have undergone a hybrid VATS.

Petersen and colleagues[4] reviewed the outcomes of 97 patients who received induction therapy followed by lobectomy from 1996 to 2005. They compared 12 patients who underwent VATS lobectomy (8 received induction chemoradiotherapy, whereas 4 received chemotherapy alone) with 85 who underwent open lobectomy. Their criteria for being considered for the VATS approach included tumors less than 6 cm in diameter, lack of airway or chest wall invasion, and no evidence of multistation lymph node disease before induction therapy. No significant differences were seen between the groups with regard to baseline demographics, pulmonary function, comorbidities, performance status, T stage, N stage, or pathologic stage. Patients in the VATS group were more likely to have smaller tumors and a lower clinical stage. Outcomes between the groups revealed no significant difference with regard to number of lymph nodes or stations sampled, 30-day mortality, or major morbidities. In addition, they reported no significant difference in overall or cancer-free survival between the groups at 2 years. However, patients who underwent VATS lobectomy had a significantly shorter median length-of-stay (3.5 vs 5.0 days) and shorter chest tube duration (2 vs 4 days). One (8%) conversion to thoracotomy was seen because of chest wall involvement.

From a series of 180 patients who underwent VATS lobectomy or sublobar resection, Shaw and colleagues[5] reported on 10 patients who underwent VATS resection after induction chemoradiotherapy for stage III disease. Of the patients who underwent induction chemoradiotherapy, no patients died, whereas 3 had only minor complications (1 with vocal cord paralysis and 2 with atrial arrhythmias). However, the extent of surgery (lobar vs sublobar) these patients received was not made clear.

The feasibility and safety of VATS resection for locally advanced lung cancer has also been demonstrated in 2 more recent studies. Hennon and colleagues[6] reported on 114 patients who were considered for VATS lobectomy. All of the patients in their series had tumors that were 4 cm or more and/or underwent neoadjuvant therapy (20%). Ultimately, 19 (17%) patients required conversion to an open thoracotomy. Of the 95 patients who underwent VATS lobectomy, the authors reported morbidity and mortality rates of 39% and 1%, respectfully. Unfortunately they did not report morbidity and mortality rates specifically for patients who underwent VATS lobectomy after induction therapy. In addition, they failed to report what type of neoadjuvant therapy the patients received.

Similar results were published by Nakanishi and colleagues,[7] who reported on a series of 76 patients (16% received induction therapy) who underwent VATS anatomic resection for locally advanced lung cancer. Locally advanced tumors were defined as central tumors that demonstrated either "a part or a whole of the lesion directly visible using bronchoscopy in the area between the mainstem bronchus and the orifice of the subsegmental bronchus, or an indirect sign caused by the lesion, such as endobronchial stenosis or extrinsic bronchial compression, was observed in the same area, although the lesion was invisible under bronchoscopic examination."[7] They reported a conversion rate of only 3%. The authors reported morbidity and mortality rates of 36% and 3%, respectively. Once again, however, the authors did not stratify their outcomes based on those that had and had not received neoadjuvant therapy.

PATIENT SELECTION

Conclusions regarding the safety and efficacy regarding VATS lobectomy after induction therapy cannot currently be made based on the existing literature. Reporting on the application of a minimally invasive approach to lobectomy after induction therapy is confounded by low numbers and heterogeneous patient populations. The authors' practice is to routinely stage patients with mediastinoscopy for any tumor greater than 2 cm regardless of positron emission tomography/computed tomography (PET/CT) findings. Patients with negative mediastinoscopy findings, including those with left upper lobe tumors and a clinically positive lymph node at station 5 or 6 based on PET/CT, are offered primary surgery. Patients who are found to have nonbulky N2 disease are referred for chemotherapy alone. Patients with more macroscopic or multistation N2 disease are referred for neoadjuvant chemoradiation, whereas those with bulky multistation N2 disease and N3 disease are considered for definitive chemoradiation. After neoadjuvant therapy, patients are restaged with PET/CT and considered for surgery if they show no signs of disease progression. Among patients treated with induction chemotherapy alone, those whose disease progresses after neoadjuvant chemotherapy or those found to have persistent N2 disease after resection are referred for radiation therapy.

There are a few clinical scenarios for which the authors do not believe a VATS approach is appropriate. If chest wall involvement is seen that mandates chest wall resection, the patient will not be spared the morbidity of rib manipulation, and therefore a thoracoscopic approach is not clearly advantageous or appropriate. Likewise, the existence of calcified adenopathy in proximity to pulmonary arterial branches generally contraindicates a thoracoscopic approach because of concerns over vascular fragility. Of course, physiologic intolerance to pulmonary resection also contraindicates thoracoscopic lobectomy, as it would an open lobectomy. That said, sufficient evidence now exists to support the notion that frail and infirm patients, in particular, benefit from a less invasive approach. The diminished impact on pulmonary function associated with a thoracoscopic approach may make pulmonary resection more tolerable in compromised patients.

TECHNIQUE

Neoadjuvant chemotherapy and particularly chemoradiotherapy tend to cause perihilar fibrosis and anatomic distortion. The tissue planes surrounding vessels are often thicker and more adherent, complicating and slowing the course of hilar dissection. The dissective stresses on named structures can be accentuated if the force is not discretely applied to the tissue that must be removed to expose a particular vessel. Stated differently, the main vector of dissective force should be applied to the nodal and connective tissue and not the named structure. The demand for precision is far greater in these cases and the tempo of dissection should be slowed. The occasional "blind" passage of an instrument around a vessel carries a greater risk of vascular injury and is ill-advised. The use of cautery often causes tissue contraction and makes identification of appropriate tissue planes more difficult. For this reason, the authors tend to begin the development of tissue planes using sharp dissection. The planes are propagated with careful sucker dissection and then veils of tissue can be divided with cautery, stapler, or scissors depending on the circumstance. If at any time vascular bruising develops, conversion to an open approach should be considered. If additional vigorous dissection of adherent planes is required, this will be poorly tolerated by vessels that are already partially compromised.

The authors' approach is designed for maximal safety during hilar dissection and has been used with great success on patients who have undergone induction therapy.[8] They typically use 4 ports.

The first port placed is typically in the midclavicular line in the fifth or sixth intercostal space; this is designated the anterior incision, meaning that it is typically at the anterior base of the major fissure and is meant to be approximately 1 inch in length. After demonstrating that the pleural space is uncomplicated, a 5-mm incision is made in the midclavicular line and the eighth intercostal space is angled upward. This location is where the camera with a 30° lens will be placed and will allow inspection for precise determination of ideal port placement for the remaining 2 ports. Note, this port is the only one that actually receives a thoracoscopic sleeve port. The authors otherwise pass the instruments in and out directly without ports. The authors' impression has been that the placement of sleeve ports to maintain site access not only limits the type of instruments that can be used but also further traumatizes the intercostal nerve and leads to postoperative neuralgia more frequently. After placing the anterior port and the camera port, the utility incision is then placed. This incision is typically at the level of the upper lobe vein for upper lobectomies and one interspace lower for middle and lower lobectomies. A tendency exists for this incision to be placed too low, which makes dissection, particularly at upper aspects of the hilum, exceedingly difficult. Therefore, the hilum should be visualized and the target site palpated for incision placement while achieving a panoramic view; this will allow the surgeon to place the incision at the appropriate level. If doubt remains, the needle used for injecting local anesthetic can be used to aid in localization before the utility incision is made. The fourth port is placed over the auscultatory triangle. It allows maximum freedom of movement through the different ports and is separated enough from the other incisions that the instrumentation will not fight for domain during retraction and dissection. This incision need be no longer than 1.5 cm to admit either a stapler or a ringed forceps for retraction. As experience grows, this incision can be eliminated. However, this teaching or assistant port allows a straight axis approach to nearly all hilar structures. Control of the operation is effectively managed through this incision.

Although in many open approaches the pulmonary vein is taken first, this consistently occurs in all VATS techniques, particularly with regard to upper and middle lobectomies on the right and upper lobe resections on the left. This technique will enhance exposure consistently to the underlying bronchus and arterial structures. This procedure is not necessarily intuitive, but with VATS such an anterior to posterior approach toward sequential hilar structure isolation is essential for safe and efficient dissection. When approaching the left upper lobe, this then allows ready exposure of the first 2 to 3 arterial branches to the upper lobe. On the right this provides immediate exposure of the superior arterial trunk. Likewise, the middle lobe bronchus is readily revealed after taking the middle lobe vein.

To provide optimal lobar retraction that separates and exposes hilar structures selectively, one must create discrete lobar separation. It is advisable very early during the VATS lobectomy to complete at least partially the anterior aspects of the pulmonary fissures. For example, when attempting a right upper lobe resection, it is highly desirable to perform 2 to 3 firings of a stapler to complete the anterior part of the horizontal fissure. Having done so, inferior and posterior retraction of the middle lobe and posterior retraction of the upper lobe allow the venous drainage from the middle and upper lobes to rotate independently; the middle lobe vein rotates posteriorly, thereby protecting it while the upper lobe venous drainage is dissected and prepared for legation and division. When approaching the left upper lobe, the lingula is typically anterior, particularly in relation to the anterior dissection port. Therefore, the anterior aspect of the fissure presents itself early for partial completion. After dividing the upper lobe vein, exposure of the bronchus and subsequently the lingular artery is virtually impossible if the fissure has not been completed. Particularly with lungs that are somewhat noncompliant and occasionally incompletely collapsed, lobar separation through completion of pulmonary fissures allows optimal retraction and selective rotation and exposure of hilar structures.

Kitner dissection has been used by some to free the phrenic nerve from its investment in proximity to the pulmonary venous drainage to upper and middle lobes on the right and to the upper lobe on the left. However, this dissection technique is imprecise, may risk traction injury to the nerve itself, causes an excessive amount of bleeding, and is not likely to reveal a clean, appropriate plane of dissection without risking potential hematoma or more serious injury to the underlying structures. The authors advocate using sharp dissection with Metzenbaum scissors to minimize bleeding and optimize dissection planes. Many have recommended dissection around structures with very large right-angle clamps. Although the long foot of these instruments is desirable in its ability to reach completely around vascular structures (particularly the vein), their considerable mass reduces tactile feedback from the instruments during dissection. Therefore, a medium right angle with a blunt tip not only is safe but also provides the right balance of tactile feedback and range of dissection.

Many surgeons have tried to insinuate the anvil of the stapler behind vessels through wiggling, rotating, or overcoming resistance with direct pressure to pass the stapler. This technique is less-than-optimal and risks significant vascular injury, which may explain why rates of significant bleeding as high as 10% to 15% have been reported. The authors' preference is to dissect the tunnel cleanly with the right angle and ensure that it is large enough to accommodate the anvil of the stapler. A tie is then passed around the vessel and used as a point of retraction. This tie can be passed out through a port that is at 90° to the axis of the stapler being passed. Alternatively, the tie can be grasped with an instrument inside the chest and retracted in multiple different directions. This technique allows retraction of the vessel away from the hilum and the passage of the stapler easily under vision without excessive twisting, axial rotation, or application of undue force. This procedure not only has been proven to be safe but also allows progressive limitation of the number and size of ports used to complete lobectomies safely. In contrast to using a vessel loop, the advantages of using a braided tie are that it can be included in the stapler firing and the loose ends can simply be trimmed. Therefore it is not necessary to remove the tie during firing. Trying to slide such a tie out after the stapler is in position risks a sawing injury to the back wall of the vessel and is unnecessary. "Rehearsal" before staple replacement can be achieved with dissection of the pathway with a pediatric Yankauer to create a tunnel or space around the vessel sufficient to accommodate the stapler. One does not want to dilate the space behind the vessel with the anvil; this is sharp and excessively traumatic. It is also critical that the stapler tips are visualized by passing beyond the target structure to be elongated and divided. Passage of the stapler tip to a so-called free space is essential for the safe conduct of this operation.

When performing open surgery, emphasis is not often placed on the removal of N1 nodes before obtaining vascular or bronchial control. Because these nodes are often included with the specimen, they are typically not taken out separately before planned lobectomy. In VATS lobectomy, performance of regional lymphadenectomy often facilitates dissection. Arterial branch points and lobar bronchial origins are marked by clusters of lymph nodes. Removal of these lymph nodes creates obvious anatomic pathways for circumferential dissection and subsequent surgical control; this is particularly true with regard to surrounding the upper lobe bronchus on the right. One or two nodes are typically present at the angle created by the inferior aspect of the upper lobe origin and the bronchus intermedius. On the left, separation of the upper and lower lobe of bronchia is facilitated by lymphadenectomy at this juncture, but separating those lymph nodes out also often allows for creation of a tunnel that will protect the continuation of the pulmonary artery, which lies behind the bronchus. Therefore, performing a preemptive lymphadenectomy as part of the dissection technique is advisable.

To facilitate dissection of the hilar structures, several maneuvers can be undertaken to separate and elongate those hilar structures. When attempting to retract the lung anteriorly on either side, it becomes apparent that it is tethered by the investment of pleura on the posterior hilum. Through lysing this pleura widely (on the right, up and around the under surface of the azygos vein; on the left, all the way up and under the aortic arch), the hilar structures will be released and allowed greater anterior retraction and separation. This technique is particularly important when performing a right upper lobectomy, because the bifurcation between the right upper lobe bronchus and continuation of bronchus intermedius is readily identified and the tunnel around it can be almost completely created from a posterior approach after having taken the superior trunk of pulmonary artery from the anterior exposure. By reflecting the lung then back into the paravertebral space, dissection of the remaining hilar structures from the anterior approach is facilitated. If one fails to open the mediastinal pleura, surrounding the upper lobe bronchus on the right from a purely anterior approach can be exceedingly difficult, and posterior parenchymal tissue is often snared in the anvil, preventing easy passage of the stapler. During a left upper lobectomy, failure to lyse the posterior pleura will make a completion of the fissure difficult without significant risk of injury to the continuation of the pulmonary artery and will compromise visualization of the remaining arterial branches to the upper lobe.

Injury to arterial branches may occur if undue dissection stress is applied as a result of an awkward dissection sequence. Some espouse leaving an arterial branch as a last named structure to be taken. However, this risks undue retraction stress on these arterial branches and may lead to surgical bleeding. By leaving a significant portion of the fissure until last, however, the lung parenchyma itself will absorb some of that retraction stress and may prevent traction injury to any named vessels. On the left side, after taking the upper lobe vein, the first 2 or 3 arterial branches, the bronchus, and subsequently the lingular artery, only 1 to 3 arterial branches remain. Although the anterior aspect of the fissure is typically taken early to enhance exposure of the bronchus and the lingular artery, it is important to leave any remaining parenchymal bridges between the upper and lower lobes intact so that posterior/lateral retraction on the specimen will display the arteries while distributing some of that tension through the lung tissue and not just the vessel. An important added benefit of this tactic is that, by avoiding dissection in the fissure, postoperative air leaks are minimized. In the authors' experience, postoperative air leaks are infrequent when the fissure is completed only with the stapler (and not using excessive sharp dissection to accomplish separation).

REFERENCES

1. Bonomi P, Faber LP, Warren W, et al. Postoperative bronchopulmonary complications in stage III lung cancer patients treated with preoperative paclitaxel-containing chemotherapy and concurrent radiation. Semin Oncol 1997;24(4 Suppl 12). S12-123–S12-129.
2. Sonett JR, Suntharalingam M, Edelman MJ, et al. Pulmonary resection after curative intent radiotherapy (>59 Gy) and concurrent chemotherapy in non-small-cell lung cancer. Ann Thorac Surg 2004; 78(4):1200–5 [discussion: 1206].
3. Huang J, Xu X, Chen H, et al. Feasibility of complete video-assisted thoracoscopic surgery following neoadjuvant therapy for locally advanced non-small cell lung cancer. J Thorac Dis 2013;5(Suppl 3):S267–73.
4. Petersen RP, Pham D, Toloza EM, et al. Thoracoscopic lobectomy: a safe and effective strategy for patients receiving induction therapy for non-small cell lung cancer. Ann Thorac Surg 2006;82(1):214–8 [discussion: 219].
5. Shaw JP, Dembitzer FR, Wisnivesky JP, et al. Video-assisted thoracoscopic lobectomy: state of the art and future directions. Ann Thorac Surg 2008;85(2): S705–9.
6. Hennon M, Sahai RK, Yendamuri S, et al. Safety of thoracoscopic lobectomy in locally advanced lung cancer. Ann Surg Oncol 2011;18(13):3732–6.
7. Nakanishi R, Fujino Y, Yamashita T, et al. Thoracoscopic anatomic pulmonary resection for locally advanced non-small cell lung cancer. Ann Thorac Surg 2014;97(3):980–5.
8. Mulligan MS. Video-assisted thoracic surgery lobectomy. Operat Tech Thorac Cardiovasc Surg 2012; 17(2):125–42.

Extrapleural Pneumonectomy for Pleural Malignancies

Andrea S. Wolf, MD, Raja M. Flores, MD*

KEYWORDS

- Extrapleural pneumonectomy • Nonsmall cell lung cancer • Malignant pleural effusion
- Pleural carcinomatosis

KEY POINTS

- Extrapleural pneumonectomy (EPP) is a radical procedure involving en bloc resection of the lung with parietal and visceral pleurae, and usually ipsilateral diaphragm and pericardium.
- EPP was initially described in the treatment of refractory tuberculosis and is currently more commonly employed in the treatment of malignant pleural mesothelioma.
- Several centers have successfully performed EPP in the context of treatment of pleural dissemination of nonmesothelioma malignancies, including thymoma and nonsmall cell lung cancer (NSCLC).
- Patients with stage IV NSCLC caused by malignant pleural effusion without mediastinal nodal or distant metastases may be considered for EPP following induction chemotherapy.

INTRODUCTION

Extrapleural pneumonectomy (EPP) is a radical procedure involving resection of the lung, visceral and parietal pleura, and, generally, the ipsilateral diaphragm and pericardium, with reconstruction of the latter two. Historically, this procedure has been employed to treat infection (tuberculosis) and diffuse malignant pleural mesothelioma. EPP may also have a role in select cases in the treatment of pleural dissemination of nonmesothelioma malignancies, such as nonsmall cell lung cancer (NSCLC), thymoma, and other tumors.

HISTORY

Irving Sarot was the first to describe the technique of EPP in the mid-20th century, as performed at the Mount Sinai Hospital in New York City.[1] He reported individual cases and results for 23 patients whose tuberculous infection of the chest was either not amenable to or had failed other treatments, such as thoracoplasty or collapse therapy. Sarot concluded that the extrapleural dissection "extend (ed) the range of excisional surgeries," enabling safe resection even in the case of empyema and total pleural symphysis. In 1976, Butchart and colleagues[2] at the University of New Castle were the first to report employing EPP to treat patients with malignant pleural mesothelioma. Operative mortality in Butchart's series was 31% and considered prohibitive, leading many physicians to question the role of EPP in treating patients with pleural mesothelioma. Nevertheless, Butchart concluded that if the complication and perioperative death rates could be reduced, the procedure could be indicated for certain types of disease. He emphasized that appropriate preoperative cardiopulmonary evaluation and careful intra- and

Disclosure Statement: The authors have no relevant financial disclosures to disclose.
Department of Thoracic Surgery, Mount Sinai Health System, Icahn School of Medicine at Mount Sinai, One Gustave L. Levy Place, Box 1023, New York, NY 10029, USA
* Corresponding author.
E-mail address: raja.flores@mountsinai.org

Thorac Surg Clin 24 (2014) 471–475
http://dx.doi.org/10.1016/j.thorsurg.2014.07.014

postoperative management were critical to reducing operative morbidity and mortality for EPP.

In the two decades that followed Butchart's series, improvements in preoperative patient selection, intraoperative technique and anesthesia, and postoperative recognition and management of complications[3] reduced the mortality of EPP to rates under 4%.[4] Modern series describing results of EPP in pleural mesothelioma patients report postoperative mortality of 2.2% to 7%.[5–9] Currently, EPP and the lung-sparing alternative, extended pleurectomy/decortication, are considered by many to have a critical role in the multimodality treatment of malignant pleural mesothelioma.[10]

PLEURAL DISSEMINATION OF MALIGNANCY

Whereas malignant pleural mesothelioma represents a primary tumor of the pleura, many malignancies, including lung, colon, breast, thymoma, sarcoma, and others, metastasize to the pleura. Reduced mortality and morbidity of the modern EPP technique have led surgeons to explore the role of this procedure in the management of pleural dissemination of other tumors (**Table 1**). Flores and colleagues[11] reported a small series of 4 pediatric patients who underwent EPP, only 1 of whom had pleural mesothelioma.

Thymoma

Thymoma in particular has a tendency toward pleural spread, and several groups have described their experience with extended resection, including EPP, for locally advanced disease.[12] Wright described the Massachusetts General Hospital experience with 5 patients who underwent EPP for stage IVa thymoma.[13] There were no postoperative deaths and one major complication (tamponade requiring removal of the pericardial patch); 5-year survival was 53% (95% confidence interval [CI] 25%–75%). In another retrospective study, Huang and colleagues[14] reported Memorial Sloan-Kettering Cancer Center's series of 18 patients undergoing extended resection for stage IVa thymoma following induction chemotherapy, including 4 patients who underwent EPP and adjuvant radiation. There were no postoperative deaths, and 5-year survival for the group (including other types of extended resection) was 78%. Ishikawa and colleagues[15] at the Tochigi Cancer Center published another report of 11 patients undergoing similar extended resection for stage IVa or IVb thymoma, with 4 patients undergoing EPP. There were no postoperative deaths, and 5-year survival was 75%.

Sarcoma

Pleural dissemination of sarcoma is difficult to treat in general and with surgery in particular. There are only rare reports in the literature describing EPP for sarcoma. In a two-patient series (1 chondrosarcoma and 1 hemangiopericytoma), 1 patient died of disease 2 years after EPP, and the other was alive 4.5 years after EPP (and 1 year following limited chest wall resection for recurrence).[16] In a more comprehensive series of patients undergoing EPP for pleural dissemination of various malignancies, Sugarbaker and colleagues[17] reported that 10 patients with sarcoma experienced a median survival of 3.7 months. Although we offer EPP in selected healthy sarcoma patients with limited or no alternative therapeutic options, we are less enthusiastic about performing EPP for this disease.

PLEURAL DISSEMINATION OF NONSMALL CELL LUNG CANCER
Nonsmall Cell Lung Cancer Staging

Like other malignancies, NSCLC may metastasize to the pleura, resulting in malignant pleural effusion. The TNM NSCLC staging system in the Sixth Edition of the American Joint Committee on Cancer (AJCC) described malignant pleural effusion without other metastases as T4M0 or stage IIIb NSCLC,[18] with many clinicians referring to this as "wet IIIb" lung cancer to distinguish it from stage IIIb patients with contralateral mediastinal or supraclavicular nodal disease. In the Seventh edition, however, malignant pleural effusion was upstaged to M1 (M1a in contrast to M1b, which represents distant metastases) or stage IV NSCLC.[19] The International Association for the Study of Lung Cancer (IASLC) Staging Committee based this change on data suggesting the survival of patients with malignant pleural effusion was similar to that of patients with distant metastases and significantly worse than that of patients with other types of T4 tumors. Five-year survival for the 471 patients with malignant pleural effusion in the IASLC database was 2%, compared with 14% in the 418 patients with other types of T4 tumors (*P*<.0001).[20]

Mediastinal Nodal Disease

The status of the mediastinal nodes markedly affects prognosis for patients with stage IV NSCLC caused by pleural dissemination. This is supported by analysis of the IASLC data, although the staging committee did not specifically compare patients with and without nodal disease. Five-year survival for the 87 N0 patients with pleural dissemination who were staged pathologically was 24%, whereas this was only 11% for the 245-patient cohort with pleural dissemination that included those with and without mediastinal and/or hilar nodal disease.[20]

Although many surgeons have clinical experience with EPP for stage IV NSCLC caused by pleural dissemination, no one has studied this rigorously, and the reports in the literature are sparse. Swanson and colleagues[21] presented their experience with 12 NSCLC patients with malignant pleural effusion and no N2/N3 nodal or distant metastases treated between 1994 and 1997. Patients were thoroughly evaluated for ability to tolerate pneumonectomy, staged with computed tomography (CT) (chest to adrenals and head), bone scan, and mediastinoscopy, and treated with three cycles of platinum-based induction chemotherapy. Patients who showed no progression following neoadjuvant chemotherapy underwent EPP, and 7 (58%) received postoperative radiotherapy. Mortality was 0, and morbidity was 58% (n = 7), mostly atrial fibrillation with 1 aspiration pneumonia and 1 vocal cord paresis. Follow-up was too short (range 3–25 months) to draw meaningful conclusions regarding survival in this small series, but the 5 N1 patients survived a median of 24 months, and 7 node-negative patients had not reached median survival at the time of the report.

Sugarbaker and colleagues[17] presented the same institution's more comprehensive series of all patients undergoing EPP for pleural dissemination of malignancy between 1994 and 2007. Twenty-eight patients had mediastinal node-negative stage IV NSCLC caused by pleural effusion. Median survival for the 9 patients with N0 disease was 52 months, compared with 14 months for the 19 patients with N1 and/or N2 disease.

Several Japanese groups have evaluated the role of EPP in stage IV NSCLC caused by pleural effusion. The Japan Oncology Group reported results of a survey distributed to surgeons performing resection on 100 patients found to have pleural effusion or pleural dissemination at the time of thoracotomy for NSCLC, but these patients were not treated with EPP.[22] Suzuki and colleagues[23] published a series of 120 NSCLC patients with malignant pleural effusion treated with intrapleural hyperthermic chemotherapy infusion in the Japanese literature. Following induction intrapleural chemotherapy, only 8 patients who were found to be free of N2 or distant metastases were resected with EPP. Yokoi and colleagues[24] at the Tochigi Cancer Center in Japan described 11 patients who underwent EPP for NSCLC with malignant pleural effusion, including 3 patients with clinical N2 disease. There were no perioperative deaths, and complications were reported in 2 patients (hemothorax and empyema in 1 patient each). Overall 5-year survival was 54.5% (95% CI: 25%–84%), with patients with N0 or N1 disease on final pathology experiencing a 5-year survival of 67% (95% CI: 29%–100%).

CARE OF THE EXTRAPLEURAL PNEUMONECTOMY PATIENT
Preoperative Assessment

The authors consider patients with pleural dissemination of NSCLC without mediastinal nodal (N2) or distant metastases for EPP following neoadjuvant chemotherapy if restaging suggests no progression of disease. Patients are staged with head magnetic resonance imaging (MRI) to rule out intracranial metastases as well as positron emission tomography-CT (PET-CT) to evaluate other metastatic sites. Endobronchial ultrasound (EBUS) or formal mediastinoscopy can rule out mediastinal nodal disease.

The remaining preoperative evaluation concerns the patient's ability to tolerate EPP.[8] Pulmonary function tests (PFTs), including spirometry and diffusion lung capacity (DLCO), should be performed. Quantitative ventilation/perfusion scan (split function test) can quantify how much perfusion flows to the ipsilateral lung. The product of the proportion of perfusion to the contralateral lung (that which will remain following EPP) and the forced expiratory volume in 1 second (FEV_1) generates the postoperative predicted FEV_1. Although many recommend a value of at least 800 cc for pneumonectomy, the added morbidity of extrapleural, diaphragmatic, and pericardial resection make it reasonable to consider a higher target, such as 1.2L, for all but the smallest patients.[6] Both a stress test to rule out inducible myocardial ischemia due to coronary artery disease and an echocardiogram with Doppler measurements of estimated pulmonary artery pressure based on tricuspid regurgitation should also be performed. The added right ventricular strain of pneumonectomy in a patient with pre-existing pulmonary hypertension may precipitate significant postoperative morbidity and/or death. Finally, the authors routinely perform duplex evaluation of the lower extremity veins to rule out deep vein thrombosis (DVT), particularly in patients who have undergone neoadjuvant therapy, as these patients have a high incidence of occult DVT, and preoperative treatment with anticoagulation (and possibly inferior vena cava filter) may reduce the risk of fatal pulmonary embolus following EPP.

Table 1
Extrapleural pneumonectomy for pleural malignancies

Author, Year	Tumor	Number of Patients	Mortality	Morbidity	Overall Survival
Wright,[13] 2006	Thymoma	5	0	1/5 (20%) major	53% 5 y Median 86 mo
Huang et al,[14] 2007	Thymoma	4	0	Not reported	78% 5 y
Ishikawa et al,[15] 2009	Thymoma	4	0	0	75% 5 y
Bedini et al,[16] 2000	Sarcoma	2	0	0	1 patient 2 y, 1 patient censored at 4.5 y
Swanson et al,[21] 1998	NSCLC	12	0	7/12 (58%) mostly arrhythmia	Median survival not reached at 18 mo for 7 node-negative patients
Yokoi et al,[24] 2002	NSCLC	11	0	2/11 (18%)	55% 5 y
Suzuki et al,[23] 2004	NSCLC	8	0	Not reported	All patients >1 y 1 patient alive as of 39 mo
Sugarbaker et al,[17] 2009	Thymoma (n = 8) Sarcoma (n = 10) NSCLC (n = 35)	65	3/65 (5%)	29/65 (45%) including arrhythmia	Median survival: Not reached at 22 mo (thymoma) 3.7 mo (sarcoma) 16.7 mo (NSCLC)

Perioperative Considerations

From the anesthesiologist's standpoint, preparation for surgery includes the placement of routine monitors, lines, and an epidural catheter for perioperative pain control.[25] An arterial line is mandated given the likelihood of rapid hemodynamic changes, and large bore intravenous access, including a central line, is recommended. If there is any question as to the possibility of existent pulmonary hypertension, the authors recommend placement of a Swan-Ganz catheter (which must be pulled back prior to division of the pulmonary artery). Central lines should be placed on the operative side to avoid pneumothorax on the side of the ventilated (and postoperatively, only) lung. Lung isolation may be obtained with double-lumen endotracheal tube (preferred) or bronchial blocker, with the latter to be pulled back prior to division of the bronchus. Finally, the authors recommend placement of a nasogastric tube to aid in identifying the esophagus intraoperatively and to decompress the stomach postoperatively. The extrapleural dissection and division of vagal fibers extending to the bronchus often lead to mild postoperative esophageal dysmotility, and nasogastric decompression may prevent life-threatening aspiration in the early postoperative period in these patients with one remaining lung.

Postoperative Care

Surgery should be performed at centers in which surgeons, nurses, anesthesiologists, and additional clinicians providing perioperative and postoperative care are experienced with the course of patients undergoing EPP. Early recognition of subtle hemodynamic and/or respiratory changes can preempt life-threatening complications. For example, proper pneumonectomy space management can prevent fatal mediastinal shift.[26] Avoiding postoperative death mandates immediate identification of tamponade, cardiac herniation, patch dehiscence, DVT, pulmonary embolus, and other morbidity.[3] Finally, careful management of fluid status and pulmonary toilet is also critical to the postoperative care of these patients.

SUMMARY

Although originally performed on patients with refractory tuberculosis and malignant pleural mesothelioma, extrapleural pneumonectomy may be used to treat patients with pleural dissemination of other malignancies, including thymoma and NSCLC. Patients who present with stage IV NSCLC caused by malignant pleural effusion may be considered for EPP following induction chemotherapy if they demonstrate no mediastinal nodal or distant metastases and have adequate cardiopulmonary reserve. EPP for NSCLC should be performed by experienced teams at experienced centers to minimize the morbidity and mortality associated with this radical procedure. Additional prospective studies are needed to better characterize the role of EPP in the multimodality treatment of patients with pleural dissemination of malignancy, including NSCLC.

REFERENCES

1. Sarot IA. Extrapleural pneumonectomy and pleurectomy in pulmonary tuberculosis. Thorax 1949;4: 173–223.

2. Butchart EG, Ashcroft T, Barnsley WC, et al. Pleuropneumonectomy in the management of diffuse malignant mesothelioma of the pleura. Experience with 29 patients. Thorax 1976;31:15–24.

3. Sugarbaker DJ, Jaklitsch MT, Bueno R, et al. Prevention, early detection, and management of complications after 328 consecutive extrapleural pneumonectomies. J Thorac Cardiovasc Surg 2004;128:138–46.

4. Sugarbaker DJ, Flores RM, Jaklitsch MT, et al. Resection margins, extrapleural nodal status, and cell type determine postoperative long-term survival in trimodality therapy of malignant pleural mesothelioma: results in 183 patients. J Thorac Cardiovasc Surg 1999;117:54–63 [discussion: 63–5].

5. Flores RM, Pass HI, Seshan VE, et al. Extrapleural pneumonectomy versus pleurectomy/decortication in the surgical management of malignant pleural mesothelioma: results in 663 patients. J Thorac Cardiovasc Surg 2008;135:620–6.

6. Wolf AS, Daniel J, Sugarbaker DJ. Surgical techniques for multimodality treatment of malignant pleural mesothelioma: extrapleural pneumonectomy and pleurectomy/decortication. Semin Thorac Cardiovasc Surg 2009;21:132–48.

7. Flores RM. Surgical options in malignant pleural mesothelioma: extrapleural pneumonectomy or pleurectomy/decortication. Semin Thorac Cardiovasc Surg 2009;21:149–53.

8. Sugarbaker DJ, Wolf AS. Surgery for malignant pleural mesothelioma. Expert Rev Respir Med 2010;4:363–72.

9. Cao C, Tian D, Park J, et al. A systematic review and meta-analysis of surgical treatments for malignant pleural mesothelioma. Lung Cancer 2014;83:240–5.

10. Rusch V, Baldini EH, Bueno R, et al. The role of surgical cytoreduction in the treatment of malignant pleural mesothelioma: meeting summary of the International Mesothelioma Interest Group Congress, September 11-14, 2012, Boston, Mass. J Thorac Cardiovasc Surg 2013;145:909–10.

11. Flores RM, Su W, Lal D, et al. Extrapleural pneumonectomy in children. J Pediatr Surg 2006;41:1738–42.

12. Wright CD. Extended resections for thymic malignancies. J Thorac Oncol 2010;5:S344–7.

13. Wright CD. Pleuropneumonectomy for the treatment of Masaoka stage IVA thymoma. Ann Thorac Surg 2006;82:1234–9.

14. Huang J, Rizk NP, Travis WD, et al. Feasibility of multimodality therapy including extended resections in stage IVA thymoma. J Thorac Cardiovasc Surg 2007;134:1477–83 [discussion: 1483–4].

15. Ishikawa Y, Matsuguma H, Nakahara R, et al. Multimodality therapy for patients with invasive thymoma disseminated into the pleural cavity: the potential role of extrapleural pneumonectomy. Ann Thorac Surg 2009;88:952–7.

16. Bedini AV, Tavecchio L, Delledonne V. Extrapleural pneumonectomy for sarcomas report of two cases. Tumori 2000;86:422–3.

17. Sugarbaker DJ, Tilleman TR, Swanson SJ, et al. The role of extrapleural pneumonectomy in the management of pleural cancers. J Clin Oncol 2009;27:7577.

18. Greene FL. The American Joint Committee on Cancer: updating the strategies in cancer staging. Bull Am Coll Surg 2002;87:13–5.

19. Rami-Porta R, Crowley JJ, Goldstraw P. The revised TNM staging system for lung cancer. Ann Thorac Cardiovasc Surg 2009;15:4–9.

20. Rami-Porta R, Ball D, Crowley J, et al. The IASLC Lung Cancer Staging Project: proposals for the revision of the T descriptors in the forthcoming (seventh) edition of the TNM classification for lung cancer. J Thorac Oncol 2007;2:593–602.

21. Swanson SJ, Jaklitsch MT, Mentzer SJ, et al. Induction chemotherapy, surgical resection and radiotherapy in patients with malignant pleural effusion, mediastinoscopy negative (stage IIIB) non-small cell lung cancer. American Association for Thoracic Surgery 78th Annual Meeting Abstract Book 1998. Boston, May 3–6, 1998.

22. Ichinose Y, Tsuchiya R, Koike T, et al. Prognosis of resected non-small cell lung cancer patients with carcinomatous pleuritis of minimal disease. Lung Cancer 2001;32:55–60.

23. Suzuki K, Funai K, Shundo Y, et al. Extrapleural pneumonectomy after hyperthermo-chemotherapy for the lung cancer patients with malignant pleural effusion. Kyobu Geka 2004;57:1023–7 [in Japanese].

24. Yokoi K, Matsuguma H, Anraku M. Extrapleural pneumonectomy for lung cancer with carcinomatous pleuritis. J Thorac Cardiovasc Surg 2002;123:184–5.

25. Ng JM, Hartigan PM. Anesthetic management of patients undergoing extrapleural pneumonectomy for mesothelioma. Curr Opin Anaesthesiol 2008;21:21–7.

26. Wolf AS, Jacobson FL, Tilleman TR, et al. Managing the pneumonectomy space after extrapleural pneumonectomy: postoperative intrathoracic pressure monitoring. Eur J Cardiothorac Surg 2010; 37:770–5.

Carinal Resection

Alessandro Gonfiotti, MD[a], Massimo Osvaldo Jaus, MD[b],
Daniel Barale, MD[a], Paolo Macchiarini, MD, PhD[c],*

KEYWORDS

- Sleeve pneumonectomy • Carinal pneumonectomy • Lung cancer • Trachea • Airway

KEY POINTS

- Carinal resection and sleeve pneumonectomy remain rare procedures, with a higher incidence of postoperative complications compared with standard lobectomies/pneumonectomies.
- Mediastinal staging is of paramount importance in selecting patients and includes positron emission tomography, endobronchial ultrasonography, and mediastinoscopy.
- Adequate patient selection, advances in anesthetic management, and surgical technique can reduce postoperative morbidity and mortality if surgery is performed in experienced centers by a skilled team.

Videos of the different phases of a carinal resection with right pneumonectomy accessed through a right posterolateral thoracotomy; and a bronchoscopy showing the endoscopic view of a tracheal replacement associated with a neocarina, performed in a patient affected by a primary tracheal tumor involving the distal third of the trachea and the carina, accompany this article at http://www.thoracic.theclinics.com

INTRODUCTION

Carinal resection, defined as resection of the trachea-bronchial bifurcation with or without lung resection, is arguably the most demanding operative procedure in general thoracic surgery.[1,2] Its indications are rare and include less than 1% of operable non–small cell lung cancer (NSCLC) extending from the lung to the carina,[3] other low-grade malignancies, and benign diseases involving the carina. These operations are carried out in only a few centers worldwide, because of their technical complexity and the general belief regarding their limited benefit to the patient.

However, recent advances have been made, including (1) performing routine mediastinoscopy and radical lymphadenectomy, because surgery is contraindicated in massive N2 disease, (2) minimizing the risks of the most fatal postcarinal resection complications, acute respiratory distress

syndrome (ARDS), by using intraoperatively lung-protective ventilation strategy techniques, including avoiding high inspiratory oxygen concentrations, reducing the number of times the lung collapses and reexpands, multiple collapse and reexpansions, preventing hypoxic pulmonary vasoconstriction during hypoperfusion of the ipsilateral lung parenchyma or hyperperfusion of the contralateral lung, and judicious use of intravenous fluids fluid overload, and (3) ensuring clearance of secretions, including a temporary tracheostomy. These advances have reduced morbidity and mortality and improved long-term outcome of such operations, and are presented here.

INDICATIONS

Eligibility for carinal resection and reconstruction should be restricted to patients younger than 75 years, with a performance status of 0 to 1, and

Disclosure Statement: The authors have no conflict of interests to declare.
[a] Thoracic Surgery, University Hospital Careggi, Largo Brambilla 3, Florence 50134, Italy; [b] General and Thoracic Surgery, Sandro Pertini Hospital, Via dei Monti Tiburtini 385, Rome 00157, Italy; [c] Advanced Center for Translational Regenerative Medicine (ACTREM), Karolinska Institutet, Alfred Nobels Allé 8, Huddinge, Stockholm SE-141 86, Sweden
* Corresponding author.
E-mail address: paolo.macchiarini@ki.se

Thorac Surg Clin 24 (2014) 477–484
http://dx.doi.org/10.1016/j.thorsurg.2014.08.001
1547-4127/14/$ – see front matter © 2014 Elsevier Inc. All rights reserved.

thoracic.theclinics.com

lesions that extend to within the first centimeter of either main bronchi or invading the carina with no distant metastasis, and normal cardiopulmonary, liver, and renal function. Surgery is contraindicated in patients with more than two N2 nodal levels above 2R/L or N3 disease (and leave immediately afterwards).[4] However, this factor does significantly increase the postoperative morbidity and potential mortality. Preoperative findings of an asymptomatic superior vena cava (SVC) invasion or limited infiltration of the muscular wall of the intrathoracic esophagus are also not operative contraindications.[5]

Chronic steroid intake should be reduced to 5 mg/d. Specific preoperative assessments should include quantitative ventilation/perfusion scans, stress spirometry, transthoracic echocardiography, and in patients with latent or symptomatic pulmonary hypertension, a basal and vasoreactive right heart catheterization with endoluminal blockage of the ipsilateral pulmonary artery. **Fig. 1** shows the oncologic algorithm; mediastinal staging includes a thorax computed tomography scan, 2-deoxy-2-[^{18}F] fluoro-D-glucose positron emission tomography, endobronchial ultrasound-guided fine-needle aspiration biopsy, and mediastinoscopy. Precise definition of any airway

invasion must be obtained by rigid bronchoscopy, during which serial biopsies of the mucosa and submucosa within at least 2 cm of the tumor surface must be taken, as well as the contralateral tracheobronchial angle and main bronchus.

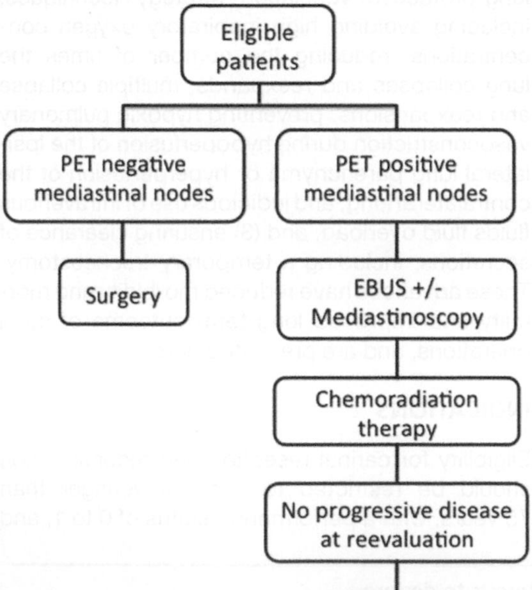

Carinal resection is more frequently associated with pulmonary resection (right or left pneumonectomy; right upper lobectomy). Rarely is it performed without pulmonary resection for lesions confined to the carina.[6] The type of resection and reconstruction depends on the location and extent of the lesion. For carinal pneumonectomy, the distance from the right distal tracheal margin to the proximal medial left main stem bronchus should not exceed 4 cm. For right-sided carinal lobectomy, any neoplasm extending more than 2 cm lower than the left tracheobronchial angle precludes a secondary end to side reimplantation of the residual bronchus into the distal left main stem bronchus. This operation should be avoided in patients with positive mediastinal nodes. Transesophageal ultrasonography can be performed to evaluate the extension of the tumor to the esophagus, left atrium, and biopsy inferior mediastinal nodes, if present. Involvement of the distal trachea and of the tracheobronchial angle is also assessed during mediastinoscopy.

OPERATIVE MANAGEMENT
Anesthesia

Total intravenous anesthesia with adjunctive epidural analgesia is usually preferred over inhalation anesthesia. Continuous monitoring of arterial blood pressure and arterial blood gases is mandatory. For right-sided procedures, patients are ventilated initially and after airway reconstruction through a left-sided double-lumen endobronchial tube. For left-sided procedures or carinal resections alone, an extralong armored endotracheal tube positioned in the right main stem bronchus or intrathoracic trachea should be used. Low tidal volume (volume or pressure) ventilation strategies techniques should be used. Careful attention to avoidance of high oxygen concentrations, reducing the number of times the lung collapses and reexpands, prevention of hypoxic pulmonary vasoconstriction during hypoperfusion of the ipsilateral lung parenchyma or hyperperfusion of the contralateral lung, and judicious use of intravenous fluids are a must. Just before airway resection, and during resection and reanastomosis, patients can be managed with the apneic (hyper) oxygenation technique,[4] as follows: patients are preoxygenated and hyperventilated with 100% oxygen (O_2) for about 10 minutes before completing the dissection to reach arterial Po_2 (partial

Fig. 1. The oncologic algorithm of eligibility to carinal resection NSCLC. Patients with involvement of more than 2 N2 nodal levels lower than station 2 and N3 lymph nodes must be excluded. EBUS, endobronchial ultrasonography; PET, positron emission tomography.

pressure of oxygen) and P_{CO_2} (partial pressure of carbon dioxide) levels of 450 or greater and 28 to 35 mm Hg, respectively. The airway is then resected while the patient is completely apneic. After completion of the resection, hyperoxygenation is initiated by placing a small (10 F) catheter across the surgical field into the contralateral main bronchus, fixing it to a cartilaginous ring (about at the 12 o'clock position) to prevent its dislocation, and connecting it to a sterile line delivering 10 to 15 L/min O_2 continuously under minimal breathing pressure (0–1 mm Hg). After reconstruction, patients are ventilated with controlled pressure through the original tube.

Surgical Incisions

Carinal resection without resection of pulmonary parenchyma and left-sided carinal pneumonectomies are approached through a median sternotomy; a combined left thoracoscopy can assist in performing the mediastinal lymphadenectomy, left inferior vein transection with EndoStapler device, and during hemostasis. With the left arm positioned in 45° of abduction, a 30° degree thoracoscope can be introduced in the left pleural cavity through a single portion of the sixth intercostal space at the midaxillary line. Right-sided lesions requiring a carinal resection with sacrifice of pulmonary parenchyma are best approached through an ipsilateral, muscle-sparing dorsal thoracotomy.

Intraoperative Dissection

Dissection must be limited to the anterior surface of the distal trachea and the first 2 cm of the contralateral main bronchus, preserving as much local blood supply as possible. Airway mobilization must be restricted to the extent needed and limited to no more than 2 cm from the proposed proximal and distal lines of transection. A complete nodal dissection is mandatory. For left carinal pneumonectomies, further exposure of the left hilum can be facilitated by using a cardiac stabilizer, applied to the apex of the heart. With concurrent use of inotropic medications, its use allows the heart to lift laterally (right) or vertically (cranially). With the heart displaced and under a direct thoracoscopic vision, the left lower pulmonary vein can be easily isolated and sectioned with commercially available EndoStaplers.

Resections

Carinal resection with right pneumonectomy/right upper lobectomy

For carinal resection with right pneumonectomy or upper lobectomy, the lung resection is the first step (Video 1). A pneumonectomy starts by dividing and securing the ligamentum pulmonalis between ligatures, then performing an extrapericardial or intrapericardial pneumonectomy in the usual fashion. Right upper lobectomy follows the same principles. To be thorough, individually secure all vessels with polypropylene sutures (Prolene, Ethicon, Sommerville, NJ). The entire right lung can then be lifted so that a complete lymphadenectomy of the lower mediastinal nodal stations can be accomplished before sectioning the airway. During this maneuver, attention must be paid to avoid damage to the left lung with excessive movement of the endotracheal tube. This goal is accomplished by gently withdrawing the tube to the level of the distal cervical trachea under the anesthetist's and surgeon's guidance. Once the tube is withdrawn, patients are preoxygenated and hyperventilated with 100% oxygen (O_2) for about 10 minutes to reach arterial P_{O_2} and P_{CO_2} levels of at least greater than 450 and 28 to 35 mm Hg, respectively, before the dissection is started. Then, under flexible bronchoscopic guidance, the distal trachea is incised with tumor-free margins, leaving the right lung/upper lobe attached to the left main stem bronchus. Next, the distal left main bronchus is resected, leaving tumor-free margins, and the right lung along with the main carina and proximal left main bronchus is removed and sent for frozen section evaluation. Frozen section evaluation is imperative throughout the operation. Ventilation is ensured via the apneic (hyper) oxygenation technique. Before reconstruction, an exploration with dissection of the contralateral nodes (4 L, 10 L) is made through the aperture generated by the resection of the tracheobronchial bifurcation.

Carinal resection with left pneumonectomy

In this case, lung resection is performed after airway dissection. After median sternotomy, the trachea is dissected, starting from the level of the innominate artery. The pericardium is opened; then the SVC and the ascending aorta are isolated and retracted laterally to facilitate exposure of the inferior portion of the trachea in the aorta-caval space (**Fig. 2**). In this phase, a meticulous mediastinal paratracheal lymph node dissection is mandatory. To facilitate carinal exposure, the right pulmonary artery is isolated and retracted inferiorly, with the left main bronchus. The right main bronchus is then exposed until the origin of the right upper lobe bronchus; the trachea is also encircled at the level of the section. Subcarinal lymphadenectomy is performed at this time. Once it is confirmed that resection and reconstruction are possible, the left pneumonectomy

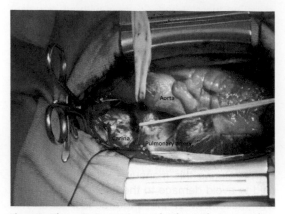

Fig. 2. The Carina exposed through a median sternotomy.

(intrapericardial or extrapericardial) is carried out. A left thoracoscopic approach can be useful not only in case of pleural adhesions but also to isolate the lower lobe vein and dissect the pulmonary ligament under direct vision. In left carinal pneumonectomy, the airway (trachea and right main bronchus) is divided and reconstructed before specimen removal. Under flexible bronchoscopic guidance, the trachea and right main bronchus are divided with tumor-free margins (frozen sections are mandatory). Although oxygenation is ensured via the apneic (hyper)oxygenation technique through the right main bronchus, the anastomosis is completed. The last step is dissection of the distal portion of the left main bronchus from the aortic arch and esophagus, so that the specimen can be removed (**Fig. 3**). Completion of lymphadenectomy and a complete hemostasis can be accomplished with the help of a left thoracoscopic view.

Carinal resection without pulmonary resection
Lesion confined to the carina: neocarina In case of lesion confined to the carina (small tumors, benign lesions [**Fig. 4**]) creating a neocarina by suturing the right and left main bronchi together and approximating these to the end of the trachea is an attractive option. This is the most anatomic reconstruction, but its use is restricted by the limited mobility of the newly created bifurcation, held down by the anatomic relationship between the left main bronchus and the aortic arch (**Fig. 5**). For this reason, the possibility for reapproximating the airway depends mainly on the mobility and the length of the trachea to the neobifurcation. As taught by Grillo, a laryngeal release does not translate to relaxation at the carina.

Carinal lesion with involvement of the distal trachea If a carinal lesion involves more than a minimal amount of the distal trachea, the remaining length of airway becomes insufficient to approximate without tension to create a new bifurcation.

In this case, several options have been described, but each one is technically demanding, associated with a high risk for postoperative complications, and therefore is rarely used.

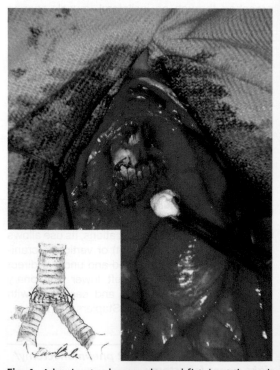

Fig. 4. A benign tracheoesophageal fistula at the carinal level. The cartilaginous wall of the airway has been opened and the fistula exposed.

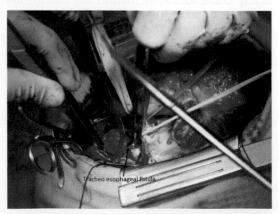

Fig. 3. Final view of carinal resection with left pneumonectomy. On the right, the specimen is exposed.

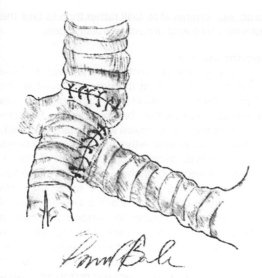

Fig. 5. A view of the final aspect of a neocarina.

1. Barclay reconstruction: end to end right main bronchus with trachea; end to side left main bronchus with intermedius (**Fig. 6**).
2. Grillo reconstruction: end to end right main into trachea; left main stem bronchus into lateral trachea.[1]
3. Eschapasse reconstruction (reverse Barclay): end to end left main stem bronchus with the trachea; end to side right main stem bronchus with the trachea (or left main) (**Figs. 7** and **8**).

All these procedures are approached via a median sternotomy and can be safely performed only in cases in which the main bronchi (particularly the right one) remains sufficiently long after carinal resection. It is easily imagined in lesions involving the distal third of the trachea that the width of airway resection is too extensive for these kinds of reconstructions. Moreover, these reconstructed bifurcations do not have an anatomic shape and consist of 2 separate anastomoses, with double the risk of dehiscence.

4. Tracheal replacement with neocarina: the newest option is tracheal replacement, whereby a tracheal graft is anastomosed to a neocarina that has been created as described, by suturing the right and left main bronchi together. The first human tissue engineered trachea replacement was encouraging and showed that such an airway with mechanical properties similar to that of the native trachea and free from the risks for rejection can be produced.[7] Video 2 shows an endoscopic view of a tracheal replacement associated with a neocarina, performed in a patient affected by a primary tracheal tumor involving the distal third of the trachea and the carina.

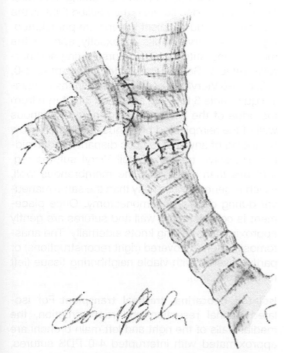

Fig. 6. Barclay reconstruction: end to end right main bronchus with trachea; end to side left main bronchus with bronchus intermedius.

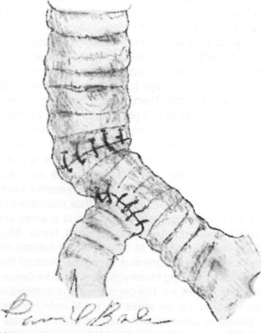

Fig. 7. First type of Eschapasse reconstruction (reverse Barclay): end to end left main with the trachea; end to side right main with the trachea.

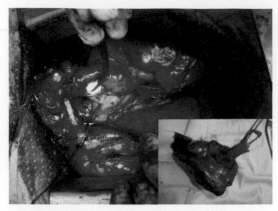

Fig. 8. Second type of Eschapasse reconstruction (reverse Barclay): end to end left main with the trachea; end to side right main with the left main bronchus.

Reconstruction Technique

General principles

The same anastomotic principles are used to perform both the end to end and the end to side anastomoses (Video 1).[4,6,8] A double-ended 3-0 or 4-0 polydioxanone (PDS, Ethicon, Sommerville, NJ) suture is started in the middle of the deepest edge of the left half of both cartilaginous walls, picking up full-thickness portions of each bronchial wall. It must be left untied to allow several stitches to be placed to complete the entire deepest anastomotic aspect and leave the membranous wall untouched. The double-ended suture is then pulled tight as the proximal tracheal and distal main bronchus are parachuted, and 2 additional PDS sutures of the same size are placed to definitively fix the parachuted suture. Consider using nerve hooks to achieve exact mucosa and stitch apposition and to avoid purse-string and narrowing effects. Then, several concentric interrupted 3-0, 4-0, or 5-0 polyglactin (Vicryl, Ethicon, Sommerville, NJ) sutures are placed on the remaining quadrants 3 to 4 mm apart and 3 to 4 mm from the airway edge. Each individual suture is positioned sequentially in a suture guide specially designed for cardiac procedures, keeping them individualized and equidistant. Once placement of all sutures is complete, the wall and sutures are gently approximated, and external knots tied. Care should be paid to avoid placing sutures on the cartilage-membranous angle, because of the high risk for tearing the airway, which can be devastating to the repair. The completed anastomosis is then tested for air leaks up to 40 mm Hg and repaired or covered with viable tissues (eg, pedicled flap of pericardial fat, pleura, or intercostal muscle). Sometimes, especially in patients who have undergone preoperative radiation, it is wiser

to accept a minimal air leak rather than to take the risks for resuturing the entire anastomosis.

Specific aspects

For carinal pneumonectomy, the end to end reconstruction starts at the deepest anastomotic edge of the left halves of both cartilaginous walls or left margin of the membranous portion. For carinal lobectomies, the choice to reimplant the residual bilobe end to side, either into the trachea or left main bronchus, depends on the length of the residual intermedius bronchus, the status of the trachea (eg, fibrotic, malacic), the extent of node dissection, and the degree of traction on residual hilar vessels. We prefer to perform the end to side secondary anastomosis into the left main bronchus.[4] During the end to side reimplantation, the residual ipsilateral pulmonary artery is always left unclamped to avoid hypoxic pulmonary vasoconstriction and hypoperfusion of the residual lobe or hyperperfusion of the contralateral lung.

The end to side anastomosis A double-ended 3-0 or 4-0 PDS suture is started on 1 edge of the deepest or posterior aspect of the anastomosis, picking up full-thickness layers of each bronchial wall, and threading the needle starting inside the lumen. It must be left untied to allow several stitches to be placed to complete the entire deepest aspect of the anastomosis before the bronchus to be reimplanted is pulled down onto the hosting structure. The double-ended suture is then pulled tight as the reimplanted and recipient lumens are parachuted. Again, use nerve hooks to exactly appose the mucosa and stitch to avoid purse-string and narrows effects. Several concentric interrupted 3-0, 4-0, or 5-0 Vicryl sutures are placed in the remaining quadrants 3 to 4 mm apart and 3 to 4 mm from the edge of the airway, leaving the membranous wall of the reimplanted bronchus until last to allow balancing of any anastomotic disparity and avoiding excessive traction. Small Vicryl sutures (eg, 5-0) are then placed on the membranous wall, which is generally less risky than the same maneuver during carinal pneumonectomy. Once placement is complete, the wall and sutures are gently approximated, placing knots externally. The anastomosis is left uncovered (right reconstructions) or partly covered with viable neighboring tissue (left reconstructions).

Isolated neocarina, tracheal transplant For isolated carinal resection and reconstruction, the medial walls of the right and left main bronchi are approximated with interrupted 4-0 PDS sutures, placed so that the knots are tied outside the lumen. Then, the anastomosis between trachea and the new bronchial bifurcation follows general principles, taking care to place the sutures proportionally in light of the size and shape discrepancy of the proximal and distal airways. Cover the neocarina and tracheal transplant anastomoses with a pedicled omentum flap (prepared through a supraumbilical minilaparotomy), or with a pedicled intercostal muscle flap, prepared at the time of thoracic incision.

Release Maneuvers

The following release maneuvers can be combined with carinal resection:

- Development of the pretracheal plane, either during mediastinoscopy or in the operative field
- Inferior U-shaped hilar release
- Pericardiophrenic release (for left-sided primary or secondary end to side anastomoses with high anastomotic tension), with separation of the pericardium and the diaphragm between both phrenic nerves.[4]

CLINICAL OUTCOMES

The 5-year overall survival after carinal resection ranges from 26% to 44% in various series.[9,10] In our experience, survival is significantly affected by endobronchial extension of the primary tumor and by nodal status (pN0 patients have a 5-year survival rate of 50%).[4] Clearly, the most important factor affecting survival is adequacy of tumor resection. The presence of metastatic mediastinal nodes in patients requiring carinal resection has always been considered a potential contraindication to surgery; we continue to exclude patients with invasion of more than 2 mediastinal nodal stations, as well as positive station 2R/L nodes or N3 nodes. Based on our previous observations,[4] for N2 patients requiring carinal resection, we recommend neoadjuvant chemoradiation, which offers several benefits: a pathologic downstaging of approximately 40%; a significant improvement of the disease-free survival after surgery; ability to undergo a more complex carinal reconstruction without significant influence on postoperative morbidity and mortality. However, some surgical oncologists still debate the benefit of induction therapy, reporting an increase in mortality after a sleeve pneumonectomy from 6.7% to 13%.[9]

COMPLICATIONS AND CONCERNS

The reported mortality after carinal resection in selected series (>30 patients), ranges from 2% to 20%. Anastomotic leaks and ARDS are the most common and dangerous complications.[10]

Acute Respiratory Distress Syndrome

In several patient series, ARDS occurs in up to 20% of sleeve pneumonectomies, with a mortality of 50% to 100%. Ventilator-induced injury and excessive intravenous fluid administration during surgery are reported as the main risk factors. Also the use of high-frequency jet ventilation has been reported as an important risk factor for development of ARDS.[11]

We suggest several precautions to reduce the risk of ARDS to be applied both intraoperatively and postoperatively:

1. Intraoperative precautions
   a. Use intraoperative lung-protective ventilation techniques
   b. Avoid high inspiratory oxygen concentrations
   c. Minimize repetitive lung collapse and reexpansion
   d. Avoid hypoxic pulmonary vasoconstriction during hypoperfusion of the ipsilateral lung parenchyma or hyperperfusion of the contralateral lung
2. Postoperative precautions
   a. Avoid hyperinflation of the residual lung
   b. Maintain adequate oxygenation with adequate pain control (with epidural analgesia or patient-controlled analgesia), chest physiotherapy, and repeat flexible bronchoscopies as needed for secretion clearance
   c. Decompressive nasogastric tube for 24 to 36 hours (to protect the residual lung against aspiration)
   d. In case of borderline predicted residual ventilatory function or reduced patient compliance, a tracheotomy at the end of surgery or in the immediate postoperative period should be considered. It also assists in secretion clearance.

Anastomotic complications

Anastomotic complications vary from granulation tissue, necrosis, mucosal sloughing, and microfistula to life-threatening dehiscence of the anastomosis.

Although chemoradiotherapy reportedly increases the risk of anastomotic dehiscence, this has not occurred in our experience. The most important factors to prevent anastomotic complications are avoidance of bronchial devascularization and a precise suture technique, without tension.

In case of an early anastomotic dehiscence after a sleeve pneumonectomy, we recommend immediate thoracostomy, because in this situation, it is critical to spatially reduce as much as possible the residual pleural cavity and control infection.

In the case of granulation tissue, partial mucosal sloughing or stricture, consider the use of a bio-absorbable polydioxanone airway stent,[12] which may offer an alternative to metallic or silastic stents as well as a definitive treatment in selected patients with airway disease, by progressively reshaping the affected airway and maintaining patency in most cases.

SUMMARY

Carinal resections and reconstructions, with or without lung resection, are challenging operations that may be indicated in less than 1% of operable patients with NSCLC or benign lesions involving the carina. These operations are completed in only a few centers worldwide, likely because of their technical complexity and the general opinion about their limited patient benefit. However, good survival results can be expected in pN0 or pN1 patients so that, in experienced hands, these operations are effective options. The risk of postoperative complications can be minimized by several intraoperative and postoperative precautions.

SUPPLEMENTARY DATA

Video related to this article can be found online at http://dx.doi.org/10.1016/j.thorsurg.2014.08.001.

REFERENCES

1. Grillo HC. Carinal reconstruction. In: Grillo HC, editor. Surgery of the trachea and bronchi. 1st edition. Hamilton (London): BC Decker; 2004. p. 599–617.
2. Grillo HC. Carinal reconstruction. Ann Thorac Surg 1982;34:356–73.
3. Mathisen DJ, Grillo HC. Carinal resection for bronchogenic carcinoma. J Thorac Cardiovasc Surg 1991;102:16–23.
4. Macchiarini P, Altmayer M, Walles T, et al. Technical innovations of carinal resection for non small-cell lung cancer. Ann Thorac Surg 2006;82:1989–97.
5. Macchiarini P. Superior vena cava obstruction. In: Pearson FG, Cooper JD, Deslauriers J, et al, editors. Pearson's thoracic & esophageal surgery. 3rd edition. New York: Churchill Livingstone; 2008. p. 1684–96.
6. Dartevelle P, Macchiarini P. Techniques of pneumonectomy. Sleeve pneumonectomy. Chest Surg Clin N Am 1999;9:407–17.
7. Gonfiotti A, Jaus MO, Barale D, et al. The first tissue-engineered airway transplantation: 5-year follow-up results. Lancet 2014;383:238–44.
8. Di Rienzo G, Go T, Macchiarini P. Simplified technique for the secondary end-to-side anastomosis in complex tracheobronchial reconstruction. J Thorac Cardiovasc Surg 2002;124:632–5.
9. de Perrot M, Fadel E, Mercier O, et al. Long-term results after carinal resection for carcinoma: does the benefit warrant the risk? J Thorac Cardiovasc Surg 2006;131:81–9.
10. Weder W, Inci I. Carinal resection and sleeve pneumonectomy. Thorac Surg Clin 2014;24(1):77–83.
11. Porhanov VA, Poliakov IS, Selvaschuk AP, et al. Indications and results of sleeve carinal resection. Eur J Cardiothorac Surg 2002;22:685–94.
12. Jaus MO, Gonfiotti A, Barale D, et al. Airway remodeling: preliminary experience with bio-absorbable airway stents in adults. Available at: http://aats.org/annualmeeting/Program-Books/2014/T9.cgi.

Lung Transplantation for Multifocal Lung Adenocarcinoma (Multifocal Lung Carcinoma)

Stefan S. Kachala, MD, Sudish C. Murthy, MD, PhD*

KEYWORDS

- Bronchioloalveolar • Transplant • Lung cancer • Adenocarcinoma • Multifocal

KEY POINTS

- Lung transplantation is a treatment option for some patients with lung-limited, multifocal adenocarcinoma.
- Preoperative tissue assessment to confirm the primary histology and mutation status and to evaluate mediastinal sites will help ensure proper patient selection.
- Multifocal, minimally invasive adenocarcinoma, even in the presence of lymph node metastases, does not necessarily preclude durable survival after double-lung transplantation in very carefully selected patients.

INTRODUCTION

Resection of early stage non–small cell lung cancer (NSCLC) provides the best opportunity for cure and remains the gold standard of treatment.[1] In patients who are medically fit with minimally invasive disease, lobar resection with mediastinal lymph node staging is the currently recommended therapeutic modality. However, there is a large subset of patients who are medically inoperable, either by virtue of poor pulmonary function or advanced disease. These patients will be relegated to wedge resection, radiation therapy, chemoradiotherapy, or palliative chemotherapy depending on the specifics of the presentation of cancer. However, there is a very small fraction of patients with a unique and rarely observed set of circumstances that are traditionally classified as medically inoperable, whose lung cancer and respiratory insufficiency can be effectively palliated through lung transplantation.[1,2]

Lung transplantation is most commonly used for the treatment of end-stage chronic obstructive pulmonary disease (COPD), cystic fibrosis, and idiopathic pulmonary fibrosis.[3] Over the course of the last decade, there has been increasing survival following lung transplantation, attributed to improvements in donor preservation strategies and postoperative critical care management.[3] New strategies for lung allocation have decreased the wait times and death rates for transplant candidates and improved efficiency within the system.[4] These strategies have allowed for an expanded recipient pool for lung transplantation, as prior absolute contraindications are being relaxed: (1) age greater than 65 years, (2) coronary artery disease, and (3) malignancy.[5,6] Although

The authors have nothing to disclose.
Department of Thoracic & Cardiovascular Surgery, Cleveland Clinic, 9500 Euclid Avenue, J4-1, Cleveland, OH 44195, USA
* Corresponding author.
E-mail address: murthys1@ccf.org

Thorac Surg Clin 24 (2014) 485–491
http://dx.doi.org/10.1016/j.thorsurg.2014.07.011
1547-4127/14/$ – see front matter © 2014 Elsevier Inc. All rights reserved.

there is still some controversy regarding these relaxed requirements, emerging data justify this practice, including some evidence to support transplantation in patients with lung cancer.[7–12]

The recommendation against transplantation in the setting of cancer stems from the chronic immunosuppression mandatory for the maintenance of the donor organ. Even in the absence of a history of cancer, chronic immunosuppression is known to increase the rates of de novo malignancy in transplant patients, with the risk of lung cancer being highest in lung transplant recipients.[13] Curiously, there are presentations of NSCLC, though occasionally widely disseminated within the pulmonary parenchyma, that have a limited invasive component and limited lymph node burden.[14] These patients can undergo a curative resection through bilateral lung transplantation and surprisingly may not possess excessive risk of cancer recurrence compared with the general population of lung transplant recipients.[11] It is paramount to appreciate the rarity of this unique presentation of NSCLC and understand when a pulmonary transplant is indicated in this setting.

PATIENT SELECTION

The selection of patients for this controversial area of lung transplantation is very stringent, as lung cancer therapy mandates the establishment of universally accepted regulations. The guidelines published in 2006 by the International Society for Heart and Lung Transplantation (ISHLT) specify absolute and relative contraindications to transplantation that could preclude a survival benefit from transplantation.[5] Most of these are common for all solid-organ transplants. Excluding history of cancer, absolute contraindications to lung transplantation include (1) a secondary untreatable advanced organ dysfunction, (2) non-curable chronic extrapulmonary infection, (3) significant chest wall or spinal deformity, (4) untreatable psychiatric condition that renders patients unable to comply with medical therapy, (5) absence of social support system, (6) substance addiction, and (7) documented noncompliance with treatment regimen.[5] Patients with untreatable advanced organ dysfunction, such as kidney or liver, lack the reserve necessary to tolerate the high-risk operation of lung transplantation. It should be noted that patients with heart dysfunction not amenable to coronary artery bypass grafting or percutaneous coronary intervention may be candidates for concurrent heart-lung transplantation.[5,6] Some chronic infections are incompatible with the required chronic immunosuppression needed to prevent graft rejection. Anatomic

deformities increase the technical difficulty of an already high-risk operation. Finally, acceptable posttransplant outcomes are tightly linked with adherence to complex medication regimens and close follow-up. Any personal or mental issues precluding recipients from actively participating in their own care should be examined in depth before listing the patients for transplant.[15]

Several relative contraindications serve to increase the morbidity of transplantation. These include (1) age greater than 65 years, (2) pretransplant mechanical ventilation requirement, (3) poor functional status and muscle wasting, (4) obesity, (5) severe osteoporosis, and (6) colonization with highly resistant organisms.[5,6] Consequently, candidacy for lung transplantation is complex and confounded by multiple independent issues. Assuming these can be appropriately adjudicated, timing and referral for listing for lung transplantation ultimately depend on the severity of the disease and the expected pretransplant mortality as well as survival after transplant.

Lung transplant candidates can expect a median posttransplant survival of 5 years,[3] and this must exceed their predicted pretransplant survival by a significant margin. The severity of disease and, more importantly, the rate of functional deterioration must be appreciated. The Lung Allocation Score (LAS) has been developed to help clinicians rank candidates based on priority. Not surprisingly, patients with the most urgent need for transplant (eg, on mechanical ventilation from primary lung failure) receive the highest LAS but are also at the highest risk for poor outcomes after transplantation.[4,16] These guidelines serve as a starting point when considering lung cancer presentations, which might allow patients to be considered for lung transplantation.

Bronchioloalveolar Carcinoma and Current Classification

In 2011, a paradigm shift in the pathologic classification of lung cancer occurred with the collaborative publication of a new lung adeno carcinoma (ACA) classification sponsored by the International Association for the Study of Lung Cancer, the American Thoracic Society, and the European Respiratory Society.[17] The most notable change from the 2004 World Health Organization classification was the discontinuation of bronchioloalveolar carcinoma (BAC) terminology.[14,17] BAC referred to at least 5 disparate tumor histologies with varying clinical outcomes and molecular properties. The new classification provides for several new entities, including ACA in situ (AIS) or minimally invasive ACA (MIA), lepidic-predominant ACA, and invasive mucinous ACA.[14] Briefly, AIS and MIA are defined as small solitary ACA with a lepidic-predominant histology that either lacks or exhibits less than 5 mm of stromal invasion in any one focus. This clinical presentation is present only in 0.2% to 3.0% of cases in Caucasian populations; but more importantly, patients with these entities experience a 100% disease-free survival (DFS) at 5 years after resection.[18,19] Lepidic-predominant ACA portends a favorable prognosis with a 5-year DFS of 85% to 90% after resection of early-stage lung ACA.[18,20] Previously, multifocal lung ACA with a limited invasive component (also known as ground-glass opacity [GGO]) had been designated as a T3/4 tumor depending on the extent of involvement; however, patients demonstrated survival similar to limited disease if complete resection could be performed.[21–24] Outcomes without resection in this cohort are very poor, with a median survival of about 1 year.[25] Finally, invasive mucinous ACA, previously identified as the pneumonic form of BAC, is distinct in its clinical, radiologic, and pathologic presentations from nonmucinous ACA.[26,27]

Mucinous ACA was an initial indication for the treatment of BAC with lung transplantation. The propensity of this histology to be multifocal and bilateral led to the reluctance to offer surgical resection as a curative option. A few patients were offered bilateral lung transplantation as the primary therapy and had reasonable outcomes.[2,7,28]

It is imperative that proper pathologic and clinical staging of such patients occurs, and this should be done in the context of a multidisciplinary tumor board in conjunction with the pulmonary transplant team.[1,11] The ideal candidate for transplantation as the treatment of lung cancer would have inoperable, lymph-node-negative, multifocal lung ACA with a limited invasive component and have limited pulmonary reserve (eg, end-stage COPD, severe bronchorrhea) that might generate LAS high enough to facilitate timely transplantation before progression of the malignancy.[1,4] The current tools for staging of lung cancer include spiral computed tomography (CT), positron emission tomography (PET)-CT, CT-guided biopsy, mediastinoscopy, and endobronchial-ultrasound. PET-CT and histology are highly predictive of patient outcomes in stage I lung ACA[29]; PET-CT assessment of GGOs are predictive of nodal status[30]; and tumor aggressiveness can be assessed using cytology alone.[31] These techniques should be used to rule out the absence of N2 disease, which is yet another contraindication to transplantation in this setting. Taken together, the presence of lung-limited ACA should not preclude lung transplantation in patients who are otherwise suitable candidates; furthermore, patients with multifocal disease should be evaluated for transplantation, which might result in a complete resection (R0) if regional or anatomic resection were not feasible.

LUNG TRANSPLANTATION
Patient Outcomes

Table 1 provides a summary of published reports on lung transplantation of patients for lung cancer. Although literature is sparse, several reports provide guidance for this narrow indication. Initial investigations sought to establish technical feasibility as well as safety. First reported in 1997, Etienne and colleagues[32] reported on a double-lung transplantation of a 41-year-old woman who presented with recurrent cancer after a previous lobectomy for BAC. Although there was no mention of objective pulmonary function, symptoms were described as dyspnea on mild exertion and chronic cough with massive bronchorrhea. Noninvasive imaging (chest X-ray, CT head/chest/abdomen) demonstrated absence of metastatic disease, pleural invasion, and regional adenopathy. Although pretransplant pathologic staging of the mediastinum was not performed, she nonetheless underwent a double-lung transplant with standard posttransplant immunosuppressive therapy. At the time of the reporting (66 months after transplant), she remained cancer free and active as a normal housewife. This patient represents an ideal candidate for double-lung transplantation, having bilateral multifocal disease, evidence of correctable functional disability, and the absence of locoregional (and systemic) disease.

This report was followed by a small case series by Garver and colleagues in 1999.[33] Seven patients were identified with stage IV BAC (multifocal and bilateral disease) but without evidence of extrapulmonary spread. No description of pulmonary function or assessment of the mediastinum was reported. Five patients received double-lung and 2 patients underwent single-lung transplantation. The recurrence of cancer was high in this series, with 4 of the 7 patients developing recurrence between 10 and 48 months after the transplant. Not surprisingly, the recurrence in 3 of the 4 patients was identical to their previous tumor as determined by molecular/genetic testing. Patient 5, who developed the most rapid pulmonary recurrence (10 months), underwent retransplantation but died just 9 months later of recurrent disease, which was still found to be restricted to the lungs (diffuse pulmonary BAC) on autopsy. In this series,

Table 1
Summary of published reports on lung transplantation for lung cancer

Author, Year	Pts	Age (y) (Mean)	Pathology	2 y OS (%)	5 y OS (%)	10 y OS (%)	Recurrence (%)	Single/ Double Lung (%)	Stage > IIIA (%)	CCOD (%)
Etienne et al,[32] 1997	1	41	BAC	100	100	NR	0	0/100	NR	NR
Garver et al,[33] 1999	7	45	BAC/DM-BAC	71	14[a]	NR	57	29/71	0	14[a]
Paloyan et al,[35] 2000	2	48	DM-BAC	50	NR[b]	NR	50	0/100	0	NR
Stagner et al,[36] 2001	2	57	Sq, ACA	50	NR	NR	100	0/100	0	50
Arcasoy et al,[9] 2001	6	59	Sq, ACA	20	NR	NR	NR	83/17	33	83
Zorn et al,[7] 2003	9	45	BMC or DM-BAC	78	52	NR	75	22/78	22	33
de Perrot et al,[28] 2004	26	44	MC-BAC	60	45	23	59	35/65	0	NR
	22	56	Stage I NSCLC	64	50	50	22	NR	0	22
Ahmad et al,[11] 2012	29	48	AIS/MIA, ACA	~62	57	25	59	21/79	14	59

Abbreviations: BMC, bronchioloalveolar mucinous carcinoma; CCOD, cancer cause of death; DM-BAC, diffuse mucinous BAC; MC, mucinous carcinoma; NR, not reported; Pts, patients; Sq, squamous.

[a] Only 1 patient had 5 years of follow-up (6 of 7 patients alive in study with follow-up of 1–5 years).

[b] One patient alive at 4 years.

4 of 7 patients still enjoyed a lengthy period of DFS (≥48 months), and 2 were cancer free at the completion of follow-up (50 and 62 months) after the transplant. This case series highlights the feasibility of this approach to diffuse AIS/MIA, but also the importance of accurate pretransplant mediastinal staging.

This same group reported on a second series of lung transplantation in 9 patients.[7] All pathology reports from previous resections were reviewed; if necessary, open lung biopsy was repeated to confirm histology. Mediastinoscopy was performed to exclude regional metastasis. Distant sites of disease were evaluated with bone scan, brain scan, CT of the chest and abdomen, and liver ultrasonography. The posttransplant 5-year survival rate was 52%, with 37% of patients experiencing good quality of life and excellent functional status over 6 years after transplantation.[7] These laudatory results are tempered by the high recurrence rate of 75%. The investigators concluded that lung transplantation can offer a strong palliative outcome in this patient population; some recurrences could be managed, but close surveillance is warranted.

A cooperative study of multiple transplantation centers reported on a cohort of 69 patients from 67 centers where cancers were identified in the explanted lungs.[28] Twenty-six patients underwent transplantation for advanced multifocal BAC, 22 of whom survived the operation. The 5-year recurrence-free survival was 35%, though actuarial overall survival at 5 and 10 years was 39% and 31%, respectively,[28] and commensurate with that expected for pulmonary transplantation, regardless of the indication at that time.[34] It was noted by the investigators that there was a higher proportion of nonsmokers in the cancer recurrence group than in the no cancer recurrence group (92% vs 44%; $P = .01$).[28]

In the remaining 43 of 69 patients with tumors in the explanted lungs, but not BAC, most patients were transplanted for end-stage emphysema or idiopathic pulmonary fibrosis. The best outcomes in this group were observed in patients with incidental stage I NSCLC; 64% of patients were alive without recurrence at a median follow-up of 30 months (range, 3–120 months). The biologic behavior of BAC in this transplant population seems to be distinct from more typical NSCLC. Curiously, for patients transplanted with multifocal BAC, the site of recurrence was limited to transplanted lungs in 88% of patients, whereas, for patients with NSCLC identified in the explant (not BAC), recurrence was universal with disseminated, systemic disease.

Two conclusions can be derived from these data. First, patients with incidental stage I NSCLC in the lung explants experience excellent outcomes. Second, despite a high rate of recurrence, lung transplantation is an option for patients with advanced, multifocal BAC. The biologic behavior of the AIS/MIA tumors seems to permit a prolonged interval to recurrence and mortality in the presence of immunosuppression.[28] The reported 39% 5-year posttransplant survival rate is promising, especially in light of the limited alternative therapies.

The most recent study used the compulsory, prospectively collected United Network for Organ Sharing database.[11] The authors sought to highlight the prevalence and clinical importance of the varying degrees of stromal invasion in the BAC tumor population. Twenty-seven of the 29 (93%) patients' pathology reports were available for review. Only 14 (52%) of the tumors were true BAC histology: AIS with lepidic growth and no foci of stromal invasion. Eleven (41%) were MIA with foci of stromal invasion in a predominant lepidic histologic background. Two (7%) patients had predominant ACA. All explant specimens were assessed hilar lymph nodes, but mediastinal lymph nodes were reported only for 20 patients (74%). Complete resection of the pulmonary tumors was achieved in 93% of patients. Patients with AIS or MIA experienced an overall survival of 57% and 25% at 5 and 10 years, respectively. Further subanalysis of survival excluding patients with ACA suggested a trend toward decreased survival with the presence of invasion, although the presence of invasion and lymph node metastases with these histopathologies did not preclude survival.[11]

SUMMARY

Lung transplantation is an acceptable treatment option in highly selected patients with lung-limited AIS or MIA. Aside from the cancer diagnosis, ideal candidates should not possess any absolute or relative contraindications to lung transplantation as described by the ISHLT. Confirmation of lung-limited disease and AIS/MIA with lepidic histology and the absence of carcinoma metastatic to mediastinal lymph nodes will optimize outcomes. Those patients with multifocal minimally invasive lung ACA and respiratory insufficiency from severe bronchorrhea may enjoy the best palliation of their disease and have high enough LAS to facilitate transplantation. The role of targeted therapies for those patients with EGFR or ALK-activating mutations and AIS/MIA has yet to be determined and might favorably impact survival and augment (or supplant) lung transplantation for these patients.

REFERENCES

1. Howington JA, Blum MG, Chang AC, et al. Treatment of stage I and II non-small cell lung cancer: diagnosis and management of lung cancer, 3rd ed: American College of Chest Physicians evidence-based clinical practice guidelines. Chest 2013;143(5 Suppl): e278S–313S.

2. Rusch VW, Tsuchiya R, Tsuboi M, et al. Surgery for bronchioloalveolar carcinoma and "very early" adenocarcinoma: an evolving standard of care? J Thorac Oncol 2006;1(9 Suppl):S27–31.

3. Christie JD, Edwards LB, Kucheryavaya AY, et al. The Registry of the International Society for Heart and Lung Transplantation: 29th adult lung and heart-lung transplant report-2012. J Heart Lung Transplant 2012;31(10):1073–86.

4. Davis SQ, Garrity ER Jr. Organ allocation in lung transplant. Chest 2007;132(5):1646–51.

5. Orens JB, Estenne M, Arcasoy S, et al. International guidelines for the selection of lung transplant candidates: 2006 update–a consensus report from the Pulmonary Scientific Council of the International Society for Heart and Lung Transplantation. J Heart Lung Transplant 2006;25(7):745–55.

6. Shah PD, Orens JB. Guidelines for the selection of lung-transplant candidates. Curr Opin Organ Transplant 2012;17(5):467–73.

7. Zorn GL Jr, McGiffin DC, Young KR Jr, et al. Pulmonary transplantation for advanced bronchioloalveolar carcinoma. J Thorac Cardiovasc Surg 2003;125(1): 45–8.

8. Sigurdardottir V, Bjortuft O, Eiskjaer H, et al. Long-term follow-up of lung and heart transplant recipients with pre-transplant malignancies. J Heart Lung Transplant 2012;31(12):1276–80.

9. Arcasoy SM, Hersh C, Christie JD, et al. Bronchogenic carcinoma complicating lung transplantation. J Heart Lung Transplant 2001;20(10):1044–53.

10. Raviv Y, Shitrit D, Amital A, et al. Lung cancer in lung transplant recipients: experience of a tertiary hospital and literature review. Lung Cancer 2011;74(2):280–3.

11. Ahmad U, Wang Z, Bryant AS, et al. Outcomes for lung transplantation for lung cancer in the United Network for Organ Sharing Registry. Ann Thorac Surg 2012;94(3):935–40 [discussion: 940–1].

12. Belli EV, Landolfo K, Keller C, et al. Lung cancer following lung transplant: single institution 10 year experience. Lung Cancer 2013;81(3):451–4.

13. Engels EA, Pfeiffer RM, Fraumeni JF Jr, et al. Spectrum of cancer risk among US solid organ transplant recipients. JAMA 2011;306(17):1891–901.

14. Travis WD, Brambilla E, Riely GJ. New pathologic classification of lung cancer: relevance for clinical practice and clinical trials. J Clin Oncol 2013;31(8): 992–1001.

15. Corbett C, Armstrong MJ, Parker R, et al. Mental health disorders and solid-organ transplant recipients. Transplantation 2013;96(7):593–600.

16. Russo MJ, Iribarne A, Hong KN, et al. High lung allocation score is associated with increased morbidity and mortality following transplantation. Chest 2010; 137(3):651–7.

17. Travis WD, Brambilla E, Noguchi M, et al. International Association for the Study of Lung Cancer/American Thoracic Society/European Respiratory Society: international multidisciplinary classification of lung adenocarcinoma: executive summary. Proc Am Thorac Soc 2011;8(5):381–5.

18. Yoshizawa A, Motoi N, Riely GJ, et al. Impact of proposed IASLC/ATS/ERS classification of lung adenocarcinoma: prognostic subgroups and implications for further revision of staging based on analysis of 514 stage I cases. Mod Pathol 2011;24(5):653–64.

19. Russell PA, Wainer Z, Wright GM, et al. Does lung adenocarcinoma subtype predict patient survival?: a clinicopathologic study based on the new International Association for the Study of Lung Cancer/American Thoracic Society/European Respiratory Society international multidisciplinary lung adenocarcinoma classification. J Thorac Oncol 2011;6(9): 1496–504.

20. Warth A, Muley T, Meister M, et al. The novel histologic International Association for the Study of Lung Cancer/American Thoracic Society/European Respiratory Society classification system of lung adenocarcinoma is a stage-independent predictor of survival. J Clin Oncol 2012;30(13):1438–46.

21. Gu B, Burt BM, Merritt RE, et al. A dominant adenocarcinoma with multifocal ground glass lesions does not behave as advanced disease. Ann Thorac Surg 2013;96(2):411–8.

22. Port JL, Korst RJ, Lee PC, et al. Surgical resection for multifocal (T4) non-small cell lung cancer: is the T4 designation valid? Ann Thorac Surg 2007;83(2): 397–400.

23. Tsutani Y, Miyata Y, Nakayama H, et al. Appropriate sublobar resection choice for ground glass opacity-dominant clinical stage IA lung adenocarcinoma: wedge resection or segmentectomy. Chest 2013; 145(1):66–71.

24. Ebright MI, Zakowski MF, Martin J, et al. Clinical pattern and pathologic stage but not histologic features predict outcome for bronchioloalveolar carcinoma. Ann Thorac Surg 2002;74(5):1640–6 [discussion: 1646–7].

25. Breathnach OS, Ishibe N, Williams J, et al. Clinical features of patients with stage IIIB and IV bronchioloalveolar carcinoma of the lung. Cancer 1999;86(7): 1165–73.

26. Awaya H, Takeshima Y, Yamasaki M, et al. Expression of MUC1, MUC2, MUC5AC, and MUC6 in

atypical adenomatous hyperplasia, bronchioloalveolar carcinoma, adenocarcinoma with mixed
subtypes, and mucinous bronchioloalveolar carcinoma of the lung. Am J Clin Pathol 2004;121(5):
644–53.

27. Casali C, Rossi G, Marchioni A, et al. A single
institution-based retrospective study of surgically
treated bronchioloalveolar adenocarcinoma of the
lung: clinicopathologic analysis, molecular features,
and possible pitfalls in routine practice. J Thorac
Oncol 2010;5(6):830–6.

28. de Perrot M, Chernenko S, Waddell TK, et al. Role
of lung transplantation in the treatment of bronchogenic carcinomas for patients with end-stage
pulmonary disease. J Clin Oncol 2004;22(21):
4351–6.

29. Kadota K, Colovos C, Suzuki K, et al. FDG-PET SUVmax
combined with IASLC/ATS/ERS histologic classification
improves the prognostic stratification of patients with
stage I lung adenocarcinoma. Ann Surg Oncol 2012;
19(11):3598–605.

30. Tsutani Y, Miyata Y, Nakayama H, et al. Prediction of
pathologic node-negative clinical stage IA lung
adenocarcinoma for optimal candidates undergoing
sublobar resection. J Thorac Cardiovasc Surg 2012;
144(6):1365–71.

31. Kadota K, Suzuki K, Kachala SS, et al. A grading
system combining architectural features and mitotic
count predicts recurrence in stage I lung adenocarcinoma. Mod Pathol 2012;25(8):1117–27.

32. Etienne B, Bertocchi M, Gamondes JP, et al. Successful double-lung transplantation for bronchioal-
veolar carcinoma. Chest 1997;112(5):1423–4.

33. Garver RI Jr, Zorn GL, Wu X, et al. Recurrence of
bronchioloalveolar carcinoma in transplanted lungs.
N Engl J Med 1999;340(14):1071–4.

34. Trulock EP, Edwards LB, Taylor DO, et al. The Registry of the International Society for Heart and Lung
Transplantation: twentieth official adult lung and
heart-lung transplant report–2003. J Heart Lung
Transplant 2003;22(6):625–35.

35. Paloyan EB, Swinnen LJ, Montoya A, et al. Lung
transplantation for advanced bronchioloalveolar carcinoma confined to the lungs. Transplantation 2000;
69(11):2446–8.

36. Stagner LD, Allenspach LL, Hogan KK, et al. Bronchogenic carcinoma in lung transplant recipients.
J Heart Lung Transplant 2001;20(8):908–11.

Index

Thorac Surg Clin 24 (2014) 493–495
http://dx.doi.org/10.1016/S1547-4127(14)00096-6

United States Postal Service

Statement of Ownership, Management, and Circulation
(All Periodicals Publications Except Requestor Publications)

1. Publication Title	2. Publication Number	3. Filing Date
Thoracic Surgery Clinics	0 1 3 - 1 2 6	9/14/14

4. Issue Frequency	5. Number of Issues Published Annually	6. Annual Subscription Price
Feb, May, Aug, Nov	4	$350.00

7. Complete Mailing Address of Known Office of Publication (Not printer) (Street, city, county, state, and ZIP+4®)

Elsevier Inc.
360 Park Avenue South
New York, NY 10010-1710

Contact Person
Stephen R. Bushing
Telephone (Include area code)
215-239-3688

8. Complete Mailing Address of Headquarters or General Business Office of Publisher (Not printer)

Elsevier Inc., 360 Park Avenue South, New York, NY 10010-1710

9. Full Names and Complete Mailing Addresses of Publisher, Editor, and Managing Editor (Do not leave blank)

Publisher (Name and complete mailing address)

Linda Belfus, Elsevier Inc., 1600 John F. Kennedy Blvd., Suite 1800, Philadelphia, PA 19103-2899

Editor (Name and complete mailing address)

John Vassallo, Elsevier Inc., 1600 John F. Kennedy Blvd., Suite 1800, Philadelphia, PA 19103-2899

Managing Editor (Name and complete mailing address)

Adrianne Brigido, Elsevier Inc., 1600 John F. Kennedy Blvd., Suite 1800, Philadelphia, PA 19103-2899

10. Owner (Do not leave blank. If the publication is owned by a corporation, give the name and address of the corporation immediately followed by the names and addresses of all stockholders owning or holding 1 percent or more of the total amount of stock. If not owned by a corporation, give the names and addresses of the individual owners. If owned by a partnership or other unincorporated firm, give its name and address as well as those of each individual owner. If the publication is published by a nonprofit organization, give its name and address.)

Full Name	Complete Mailing Address
Wholly owned subsidiary of	1600 John F. Kennedy Blvd. Ste. 1800
Reed/Elsevier, US holdings	Philadelphia, PA 19103-2899

11. Known Bondholders, Mortgagees, and Other Security Holders Owning or Holding 1 Percent or More of Total Amount of Bonds, Mortgages, or Other Securities. If none, check box   ☐ None

Full Name	Complete Mailing Address
N/A	

12. Tax Status (For completion by nonprofit organizations authorized to mail at nonprofit rates) (Check one)
The purpose, function, and nonprofit status of this organization and the exempt status for federal income tax purposes:
☐ Has Not Changed During Preceding 12 Months
☐ Has Changed During Preceding 12 Months (Publisher must submit explanation of change with this statement)

PS Form 3526, August 2012 (Page 1 of 3 (Instructions Page 3))   PSN 7530-01-000-9931   PRIVACY NOTICE: See our Privacy policy in www.usps.com

13. Publication Title	14. Issue Date for Circulation Data Below
Thoracic Surgery Clinics	August 2014

15. Extent and Nature of Circulation			Average No. Copies Each Issue During Preceding 12 Months	No. Copies of Single Issue Published Nearest to Filing Date
a. Total Number of Copies (Net press run)			713	642
b. Paid Circulation (By Mail and Outside the Mail)	(1)	Mailed Outside-County Paid Subscriptions Stated on PS Form 3541. (Include paid distribution above nominal rate, advertiser's proof copies, and exchange copies)	370	286
	(2)	Mailed In-County Paid Subscriptions Stated on PS Form 3541 (Include paid distribution above nominal rate, advertiser's proof copies, and exchange copies)		
	(3)	Paid Distribution Outside the Mails Including Sales Through Dealers and Carriers, Street Vendors, Counter Sales, and Other Paid Distribution Outside USPS®	136	144
	(4)	Paid Distribution by Other Classes Mailed Through the USPS (e.g. First-Class Mail®)		
c. Total Paid Distribution (Sum of 15b (1), (2), (3), and (4))			506	430
d. Free or Nominal Rate Distribution (By Mail and Outside the Mail)	(1)	Free or Nominal Rate Outside-County Copies Included on PS Form 3541	56	62
	(2)	Free or Nominal Rate In-County Copies Included on PS Form 3541		
	(3)	Free or Nominal Rate Copies Mailed at Other Classes Through the USPS (e.g. First-Class Mail)		
	(4)	Free or Nominal Rate Distribution Outside the Mail (Carriers or other means)		
e. Total Free or Nominal Rate Distribution (Sum of 15d (1), (2), (3) and (4)			56	62
f. Total Distribution (Sum of 15c and 15e)			562	492
g. Copies not Distributed (See instructions to publishers #4 (page #3))			151	150
h. Total (Sum of 15f and g)			713	642
i. Percent Paid (15c divided by 15f times 100)			90.04%	87.40%

16.Total circulation includes electronic copies. Report circulation on PS Form 3526-X worksheet.

17. Publication of Statement of Ownership
If the publication is a general publication, publication of this statement is required. Will be printed in the November 2014 issue of this publication.

18. Signature and Title of Editor, Publisher, Business Manager, or Owner

Stephen R. Bushing – Inventory Distribution Coordinator

Date
September 14, 2014

I certify that all information furnished on this form is true and complete. I understand that anyone who furnishes false or misleading information on this form or who omits material or information requested on the form may be subject to criminal sanctions (including fines and imprisonment) and/or civil sanctions (including civil penalties).

PS Form 3526, August 2012 (Page 2 of 3)

Moving?

Make sure your subscription moves with you!

To notify us of your new address, find your **Clinics Account Number** (located on your mailing label above your name), and contact customer service at:

Email: journalscustomerservice-usa@elsevier.com

800-654-2452 (subscribers in the U.S. & Canada)
314-447-8871 (subscribers outside of the U.S. & Canada)

Fax number: 314-447-8029

Elsevier Health Sciences Division
Subscription Customer Service
3251 Riverport Lane
Maryland Heights, MO 63043

ELSEVIER

Moving?

Make sure your subscription moves with you!

To notify us of your new address, find your Clinics Account Number (located on your mailing label above your name) and contact customer service at:

Email: journalscustomerservice-usa@elsevier.com

800-654-2452 (subscribers in the U.S. & Canada)
314-447-8871 (subscribers outside of the U.S. & Canada)

Fax number: 314-447-8029

**Elsevier Health Sciences Division
Subscription Customer Service
3251 Riverport Lane
Maryland Heights, MO 63043**

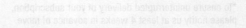

To ensure uninterrupted delivery of your subscription, please notify us at least 4 weeks in advance of move.